Fundamentals
of Mammography

Fundamentals of Mammography

3rd edition

SUSAN WILLIAMS

Consultant Radiographer
Shrewsbury and Telford Hospital NHS Trust

KATHRYN TAYLOR

Consultant Radiographer
Cambridge University Hospitals NHS Foundation Trust

STELLA CAMPBELL

Consultant Radiographer
Yeovil District Hospital NHS Foundation Trust

ELSEVIER

First edition 1995
Second edition 2003

ISBN: 978-0-702-08107-1

Content Strategist: Trinity Hutton
Content Development Specialist: Andrae Akeh
Publishing Services Manager: Shereen Jameel
Senior Project Manager: Umarani Natarajan
Design Direction: Bridget Hoette

Printed in India by Thomson Press India Ltd.

Last digit is the print number: 9 8 7 6 5 4 3 2 1

CONTENTS

Breast cancer remains one of the most common cancers in women, and early detection is essential to the successful treatment and management of the disease. In recent years, there has been a huge surge in available technologies for both the diagnosis and management of breast disease. However, high quality mammography used as a screening tool or as an assessment tool remains the backbone of the diagnostic workup for breast disease.

The aim of this book is to assist trainee and qualified mammographers in delivering a consistently high quality service. We hope to develop their background knowledge to give a better understanding of the essential role they play within the multidisciplinary team.

An understanding of not only the technical and physical aspects of mammography, but how and why the resultant images are used for the interpretation and management of breast diseases will help practitioners to make good clinical choices. This can only improve patient care and outcomes.

Technology and new models of care have seen tremendous changes in the way breast services are delivered since the original version of this book. Skill mix is now well established, and a much more multidisciplinary approach is taken to service delivery.

For the purposes of consistency and ease throughout the book, the following terms will be used to describe the practitioner undertaking any given task:

Mammographer—any practitioner that is suitably trained to undertake mammographic images. This includes radiographers (state-registered practitioners) and assistant practitioners (working under the indirect supervision of a radiographer)

Reader—any practitioner able to interpret mammographic images

A generic term of woman will be applied to any person requiring mammograms in either the screening or symptomatic setting. Please note that much of the information for symptomatic women also applies to male patients.

At the end of each chapter, a reading list is provided to recognize the international variations and commonalities in practice, which may be of interest for the reader who wishes to explore the topic further.

ACKNOWLEDGEMENT

I would like to thank all of the people that have so generously donated their time to the completion of this book. Firstly to Ian, Sian, Lucy, Sharon, Deb, Linda, and all the people who kindly agreed to allow us to use their images for benefit of others, we could not have done this without you.

Thank you to the all companies that have allowed us to include their equipment in our images and the publishers for having faith in us.

Thanks to Kathryn for agreeing to share the load. A special thank you to Stella for helping us get the book completed on time, your contribution has been invaluable.

We have got to know each other pretty well over recent months having spent almost every day going over the chapters. The experience has been both rewarding and enlightening; it has been a pleasure and I hope the reader finds the content both practical and useful. Enjoy.

Susan Williams

AEC	automatic exposure control	MRI	magnetic resonance imaging
AI	artificial intelligence	MWL	modality worklist
AP	advanced practitioner	NBSS	National Breast Screening Services
AWS	acquisition workstation	NHS	National Health Service
CAD	computer-aided diagnosis	NHSBSP	National Health Service Breast Screening Programme
CC	craniocaudal		
CNR	contrast-to-noise ratio	PACS	picture archiving and communication system
DBT	digital breast tomosynthesis	PHE	Public Health England
DCIS	ductal carcinoma in situ	QA	quality assurance
DICOM	Digital Imaging and Communication in Medicine	RA	responsible assessor
		RIS	radiology information system
EPR	electronic patient record	ROI	region of interest
FFDM	full-field digital mammography	RQAS	Regional Quality Assurance Service
HIS	hospital information system	SCoR	Society and College of Radiographers
HRT	hormone replacement therapy	SD	standard deviation
IEP	image exchange portal	SNLB	sentinel lymph node biopsy
IR(ME)R	ionizing radiation (medical exposure) regulations	SMPTE	Society of Motion Picture and Television
		SNR	signal-to-noise ratio
kVp	kilo voltage peak	SQAS	screening quality assurance service
LAN	local area network	TDLU	terminal duct lobule unit
LBD	light beam diaphragm	TR/TP	technical repeat/recall
LCIS	lobular carcinoma in situ	TQM	total quality management
M	mean	US	ultrasound
mAs	milliamperage/second	VAB	vacuum-assisted biopsy
MDT	multidisciplinary team	VAE	vacuum-assisted excision
MLO	mediolateral oblique	WAN	wide area network

Fundamentals
of Mammography

Mammography Equipment and Quality Control

CHAPTER CONTENTS

OBJECTIVES

This chapter outlines:
- The basic requirements of mammography equipment
- Routine quality control testing

INTRODUCTION

The purchase, commissioning and quality control of equipment is essential to the provision of a quality mammographic service. It is essential that the equipment is fit for purpose otherwise the technical expertise of the mammographer will be wasted and the diagnostic information available to correctly interpret resultant images reduced. Mammography requires the highest image quality of all x-ray procedures. The use of dedicated equipment with high specifications used by highly trained experts leads to maximum visibility of breast anatomy and signs of pathology.

MAMMOGRAPHIC EQUIPMENT CHOICE

Design

The equipment chosen for mammography must be acceptable to both the mammographer and the woman to be examined and able to produce consistent quality images at high volume. It must be easy to use and, especially in the screening situation, should be light to manipulate. Large, unwieldy equipment is usually physically demanding on the mammographers who have to use it, and to this end, its ergonomic design is all important. Most modern equipment is designed with women in mind in terms of esthetic appearance. All areas of the equipment which come into contact with the woman must be smooth, with no sharp edges or corners, and no external parts should become excessively hot.

Most women are able to stand while mammography is performed, but handles must be available at appropriate levels to allow the unsteady or frail to hold on without compromising the accurate positioning of the breast and adjacent pectoralis major muscle.

The perfect mammography unit has not yet been designed from the point of view of either the mammographer or the woman. Some designs are better than others, but choosing equipment always involves compromise. In the United Kingdom, as part of the breast screening program, most x-ray units have been independently tested and evaluated to help potential buyers select the unit that best meets their needs.

The basic mammography equipment consists of: a control console with radiation shield and monitor, a generator, upright gantry, capable of angulation, an x-ray tube, x-ray filter, collimator, detector plates, automatic exposure device, compression paddles, face guard, handles, foot and hand control controls for compression and height adjustment, manual compression controls (Fig. 1.1).

Functional Requirements

It is important that the machine is able to perform to a consistently high standard over time. Very small changes in the breast may be the only indication that there is a developing cancer. Mammography provides a mechanism for early detection, but the equipment must be reliable and consistent in its performance. It should be robust enough to cope with in excess of 300 exposures per day. Most full field

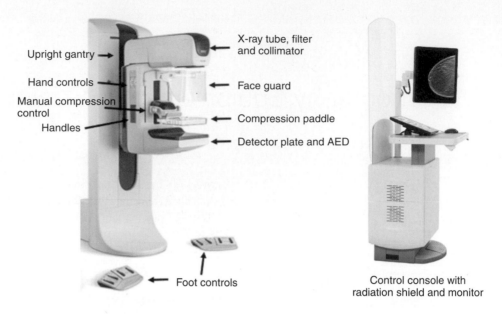

Fig. 1.1 Basic mammography equipment. Courtesy of Hololologic Inc.

digital mammography systems consist of a digital detector with a range of compression paddles and accessories allowing a full range of mammographic techniques.

The mammography unit will generally have an associated acquisition workstation, which provides a limited range of image processing functions, a display system on which to review the acquired images, and a system on which to store, archive, and retrieve images.

The following equipment parameters must be considered:

Electricity supply

Any x-ray equipment has to meet requirements with regard to supply, connectivity, and safety. Although some of these requirements are applicable to all equipment, there may be variations between manufacturers and models that need to be considered. Whether the unit is to be used in a static unit or on a mobile trailer should be considered. The supplier is responsible for electrical provision, and the owner has the responsibility for the safety of staff and women under the Health and Safety at Work Act 1974. The power supply should be uninterrupted.

Acquisition system

The mammography unit generates x-rays which penetrate the breast tissue to reach the image receptor (detector). Detectors have a range of technologies available dependent on the manufacturer. All of them will convert radiation into an electronic format in a slightly different way and will each have inherent strengths and weaknesses associated with their respective systems. The detector has a wide dynamic range which provides the opportunity for the mammographer to manipulate the image and enhance contrast characteristics.

X-ray generator and tube

The tube has a low energy x-ray spectrum of between 24 and 35 kVp in 1 kVp steps to emphasis compositional differences of the breast. They have dual focal spot sizes of 0.3 for routine mammography and 0.1 for magnification views. The focus image distance is generally in the range of 60 to 65 cm. The tube current (mA) should be as high as possible, at least 5 to 400 mA, and an exposure time range of 30 ms to 2 s to minimize the risk of movement blur.

Automatic exposure control (AEC)

An accurate AEC device is essential. The AEC system measures the radiation reaching the detector and terminates the exposure when the necessary radiation has been delivered to produce the expected density image. Digital units use superpixel technology to determine the optimum exposure factors for any breast density. The AEC is calibrated by engineers to produce the optimum density for the specific clinical setting. The unit should allow the mammographer to override the AEC and set manual exposures.

Grid

An antiscatter grid is used in digital mammography to reduce the scattered radiation from the breast and to improve image quality.

Acquisition workstation (AWS)

The AWS is usually near the mammography unit, the monitor is not suitable for interpreting the images but will allow the mammographer to review the technical quality of mammography images, input information, and apply a limited range of postprocessing applications. The information about the image from the detector will automatically be processed by the application of a suitable algorithm before it is displayed on the monitor. The mammographer may be able to select an alternative postprocessing option to optimize the image depending on the examination and projection.

POSTINSTALLATION PROCEDURES

A critical inspection, carried out by competent, qualified engineers, is mandatory to ensure that the equipment has been delivered and installed according to specification and to confirm complete electrical safety. Independent, quality control, medical physicists must then carry out commissioning and acceptance tests. These tests should follow clearly defined and recognized guidelines, such as those defined by the UK's Institute of Physics and Engineering in Medicine.

Before any mammography is undertaken, a mammographer should check that the equipment is functioning satisfactorily and that it is safe. A radiographer, at commissioning, and at regular intervals, should carry out the following safety checks thereafter.

- There should be no sharp edges
- The emergency power switch should work quickly and easily.
- The compression should be released on emergency switch-off.
- There should be no powered movement of the detector plate when compression is applied
- There should be the capability to override the automatic release of compression after exposure
- The maximum compression force should be limited to 200 newtons (20 kg).
- The light within the light beam diaphragm (LBD) should remain on for no longer than 120 seconds, and the area surrounding the LBD should not feel unduly hot to the woman, should she come into contact with it.
- All mechanical movements should be free running, and all brakes should function correctly. There should be no overrun of any movement following release of the drive switch.
- All accessories should attach easily and securely. There should be no risk of injury to the mammographer or to the woman being examined.

ROUTINE SYSTEMS CHECKS

Before testing, the equipment should be warmed up according to the manufacturer's instructions. A range of daily, weekly, and monthly tests are used to manage the attainment of consistent image quality. A set of routine user tests are indicated to detect changes in the performance of the x-ray unit or the image receptor. Each department should have detailed instructions for staff regarding when and how to perform the test and the actions to take if the results indicate a potential problem.

Equipment Required for Quality Control Testing of the Mammography System

- Perspex block 4 or 4.5 cm thick; this mimics the absorption of the "standard" breast, further blocks can be used to simulate thicker breasts (Fig. 1.2).

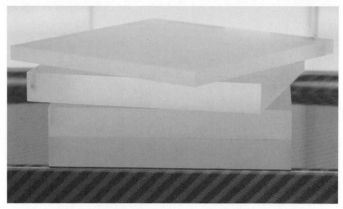

Fig. 1.2 Perspex blocks for quality control tests.

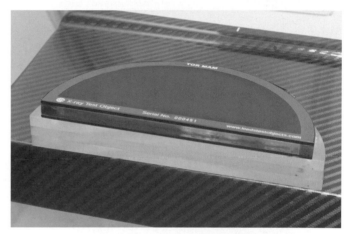

Fig. 1.3 An image quality phantom.

- 0.2 mm piece of aluminum foil (AL) fixed between the Perspex with one edge of the midline, image quality phantom (Fig. 1.3).

In the United Kingdom, the National Health Service Breast Screening Programme (NHSBSP) recommends the following.

Daily Systems Check

This test should be performed the same way every day using Perspex blocks and an AL square as shown in Fig. 1.4. A dedicated compression paddle should be used. The block is placed on the detector and the compression plate lowered to a consistent thickness or compression force. An automatic exposure is used, and the exposure factors and dose to the detector recorded. The image should be examined for artefacts using a narrow window width. A region of interest (ROI) (see Fig. 1.4) and the mean (M) and standard deviation (SD) of the pixel value or the signal-to-noise ratio (SNR) is identified; the SNR is also obtained by the equation SNR = M/SD. The SNR is the relative contribution of useful signals and random superimposed signals (background noise). Subsequent readings should be within 10% of the baseline recordings.

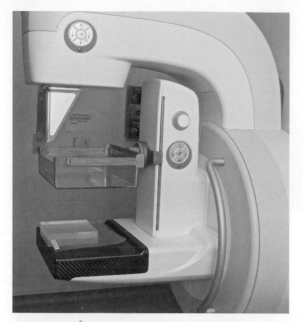

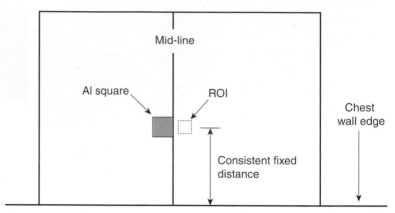

Fig. 1.4 Region of interest for signal-to-noise ratio measurement.

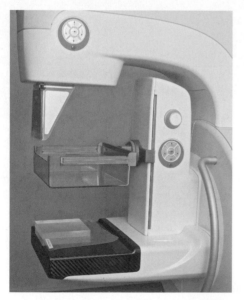

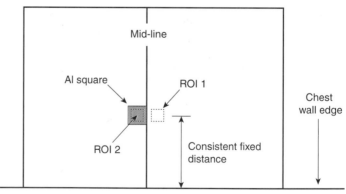

Fig. 1.5 Region of interest for contrast-to-noise ratio measurement.

Weekly Check of Contrast-to-Noise Ratio

Equipment is set up as seen in Fig. 1.5. Using the daily image, a second ROI is drawn over the aluminum foil and the mean pixel value is recorded (M1). Contrast-to-noise ratio (CNR) = M−M1/SD. Subsequent readings should be within 10% of the baseline recordings (see Fig. 1.5). Contrast-to-noise is the ability to visualize different tissues through background noise.

To check the AEC device, the SNR and CNR tests should be repeated on different thicknesses of Perspex on a monthly basis.

Weekly Artefact and Uniformity Check

It is important all components are clean before performing this test and set up as in Fig. 1.6. The image should be inspected systematically to look for artefacts like blurring or faulty pixels. The uniformity test, with the appropriate tool (see Fig. 1.6) should be repeated for all target/filter combinations used clinically. The test should follow as per the daily test but using multiple ROIs (see Fig. 1.6) on the first image. The mean pixel value should be recorded for the ROIs, the central ROI, and the one with the greatest difference, these values should be used to calculate the

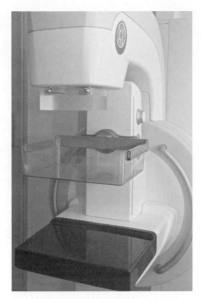

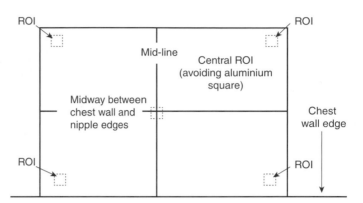

ROI   ROI

Mid-line

Central ROI
(avoiding aluminium
square)

Midway between
chest wall and
nipple edges

Chest
wall edge

ROI   ROI

Fig. 1.6 Region of interest for uniformity check.

maximum percentage deviation, which should be no more than 10%.

Testing Image Quality

Image quality should be checked using an image quality test phantom (see Fig. 1.3). This test will assess the whole system, including the imaging system. The test object should be used according to the manufacturer's instruction manual. An image should be taken weekly of the image test phantom (Fig. 1.7)

and compared with the "gold standard" agreed documented standards. The test should be repeated following any servicing or repair of the equipment or when a problem is suspected.

Appropriate tests should be carried out after a mobile unit has moved. There should be clear handover procedures with engineers and medical physicists and appropriate tests performed after an engineer's visit or changes to any part of the imaging chain (x-ray unit, software, workstations, etc.).

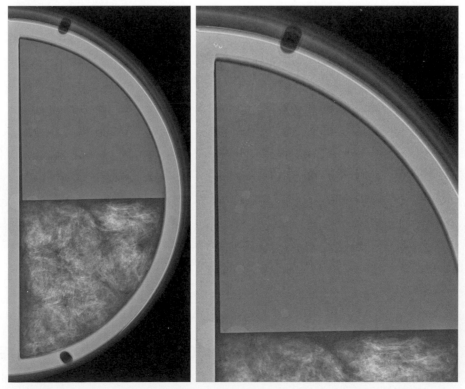

Fig. 1.7 Radiographic image of the image quality phantom—normal and close up.

DIGITAL BREAST TOMOSYNTHESIS

Digital breast tomosynthesis (DBT) is a newly developed form of imaging the breast that results in a three-dimensional image, improving the accuracy of mammography because of a reduction in tissue overlap. Multiple images of the breast are acquired at different angles of the x-ray tube. The images can then be viewed sequentially to allow the viewer to look at slices through the breast, rather than the whole breast at once.

To enable this technology to work, manufacturers have made adaptations to the x-ray unit to allow higher energy spectrums using different materials for both the targets and filters. The way the machine moves and the number of projections are influenced by a number of factors including scan time, electronic noise, and tube angle.

DBT has its own set of quality assurance (QA) tests, including adaptations of the tests for the standard two-dimensional x-ray unit.

STEREOTACTIC DEVICES

Stereotactic devices, if seldom used, should be tested before each use or weekly if in constant use. This is carried out using a dedicated test object which usually consists of a plastic block with pins at varying distances from the detector plate. These are generally supplied by the equipment manufacturer (Fig. 1.8).

Testing Stereotactic Devices

The stereotactic device is installed according to the manufacturer's instructions. The test object is placed on the detector plate in the position that the breast would occupy. An initial scout exposure will be required. Two exposures are made with the tube angled through 15 degrees to either side (Fig. 1.9), according to the manufacturer's instructions. Following the instructions pertinent to the equipment, the device is localized. The needle guide is placed in the position required to target the identified area. The needle is selected from the menu at the acquisition workstation and checked for accuracy (Fig. 1.10). All types of needles listed in the

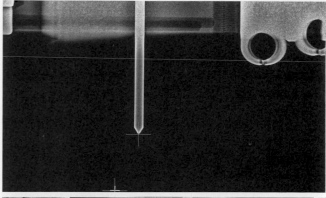
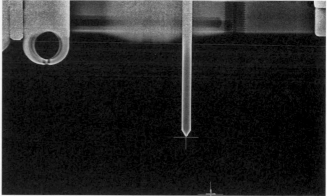

Fig. 1.9 Stereotactic pair for testing the accuracy of targeting for localization procedures.

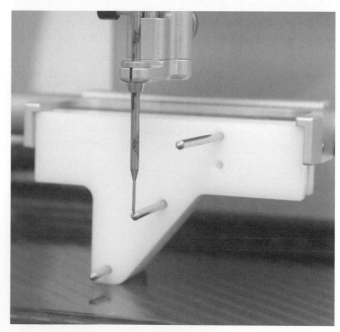

Fig. 1.10 Accuracy of the targeted lesion and needle selected.

menu should be tested on a regular basis. Needles no longer used at the facility should be removed from the menu.

DOCUMENTING TEST RESULTS

The checks should be recorded in a standard format so trends and problems can be easily identified and actioned (Fig. 1.11).

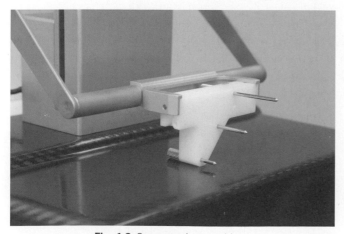

Fig. 1.8 Stereotactic test object.

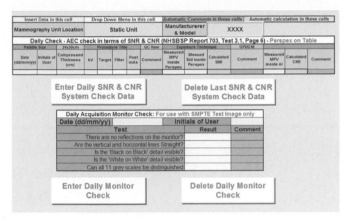

Fig. 1.11 Routine quality assurance tests database for mammography equipment.

FURTHER READING

Moustafa, A. (2013). Features of modern mammography equipment. Available at: doi: 10.13140/RG.2.2.20473.47207. (Accessed 17/04/20).

Amendoeira, I., Perry, N., Broeders, M., et al. (2013). *European guidelines for quality assurance in breast cancer screening and diagnosis* (pp. 1-160). European Commission.

Bain, K., Howells P., Rodaks. G. (2012). *The critical examination of x-ray generating equipment in diagnostic radiology.* IPEM.

Burch, A., Hay, E., Loader, R., et al. (2014). *Routine quality control tests for breast tomosynthesis (Radiographers).* (NHSBSP Equipment Report 1406). Sheffield: NHS Cancer Screening Programmes. Available at: https://assets.publishing.service.gov.uk/government/uploads/system/uploads/attachment_data/file/442730/nhsbsp-equipment-report-1406.pdf (Accessed 16/04/20).

Department of Health and Social Care. (2017). *Guidance to the ionising radiation (medical exposure) regulations 2017.* gov.uk. Available at: https://www.gov.uk/government/publications/ionising-radiation-medical-exposure-regulations-2017-guidance (Accessed 3/1/2020).

Health and Safety at Work etc. Act 1974. *Chapter 37.* Available at: http://www.legislation.gov.uk/ukpga/1974/37/section/2 (Accessed 3/1/2020).

IAEA. (2016). *Digital Mammography Unit and Associated Services, Project GE06010.* Available at: https://www-pub.iaea.org/MTCD/Publications/PDF/Pub1482_web.pdf (Accessed 17/04/20).

Kanal, K.M., Krupinski, E., Berns, E.A., et al. (2013). ACR–AAPM–SIIM Practice Guideline for Determinants of Image Quality in Digital Mammography. *Journal of Digital Imaging* 26, 10–25.

Mackenzie, A., Warren, L.M., Wallis, M.G., et al. (2016). The relationship between cancer detection in mammography and image quality measurements. *Physica Medica*, 32(4), 568–574.

Mansfield, B., Lawinski., C.P. (2012). Guidance notes for the installation of electrical supply in mobile trailers for breast screening. Publication 72. NHS Cancer Screening Programmes. Available at: https://assets.publishing.service.gov.uk/government/uploads/system/uploads/attachment_data/file/441751/nhsbsp72.pdf (Accessed 16/04/20).

Black, R. (ed.). (2012). *The critical examination of x-ray generating equipment in diagnostic radiology.* Medical Engineering and Physics (MEP). Available at: https://www.ipem.ac.uk/ScientificJournalsPublications/TheCriticalExaminationofX-RayGeneratingEquip.aspx (Accessed 16/04/2020).

NHS Cancer Screening Programmes (2009). Commissioning and Routine Testing of Full Field Digital Mammography Systems, Equipment Report 0604, Version 3 Available at: https://assets.publishing.service.gov.uk/government/uploads/system/uploads/attachment_data/file/441857/nhsbsp-equipment-report-0604.pdf (Accessed 16/04/2020).

NHS Cancer Screening Programmes. (2013). *Routine quality control tests for full-field digital mammography systems. Equipment report 1303: fourth edition* October. Available at: https://assets.publishing.service.gov.uk/government/uploads/system/uploads/attachment_data/file/442720/nhsbsp-equipment-report-1303.pdf (Accessed 16/04/2020).

NHS Cancer Screening Programmes (2014). Guidance notes for equipment evaluation and protocol for user evaluation of imaging equipment for mammographic screening and assessment NHSBSP Equipment Report 1411. September. Available at: https://assets.publishing.service.gov.uk/government/uploads/system/uploads/attachment_data/file/442723/nhsbsp-equipment-report-1411.pdf (Accessed 16/04/20).

Panetta, D., Demi, M. (2014). Introduction to volume 2: x-ray and ultrasound imaging. In A. Brahme (Ed.), *Comprehensive biomedical physics* (pp. 13–16). Elsevier.

Perry, N., Puthaar, E., Broeders, M., et al. (2008). European guidelines for quality assurance in breast cancer screening and diagnosis. Fourth Edition – summary document. *Annals of Oncology* 19(4), 614-622.

Philpotts, L.E., Hooley, R.J. (2017). *Breast tomosynthesis.* Elsevier.

Public Health England. (2017). NHS Breast Screening Programme Guidance for breast screening mammographers. 3rd Ed. Available at: https://assets.publishing.service.gov.uk/government/uploads/system/uploads/attachment_data/file/819410/NHS_Breast_Screening_Programme_Guidance_for_mammographers_final.pdf (Accessed 16/04/20).

Public Health England. (2019). *Breast screening: guidelines for medical physics services.* Breast Screening: Quality Assurance for Medical Physics Services. Available at: https://www.gov.uk/government/publications/breast-screening-quality-assurance-for-medical-physics-services/breast-screening-guidelines-for-medical-physics-services (Accessed 16/04/2020).

Reis, C., Pascoal, A., Sakellaris, T., Koutalonis, M. (2013). Quality assurance and quality control in mammography: a review of available guidance worldwide. *In Insights into Imaging.* Available at: https://doi.org/10.1007/s13244-013-0269-1 (Accessed 16/04/20).

Taibl, A., Vecchio, S. (2014). Breast Imaging. In Brahme. A. (Ed). *Comprehensive biomedical physics. volume 2. x-ray and ultrasound* (p. 121 – 154). Oxford: Elsevier.

Image Display and Storage

OBJECTIVES

This chapter outlines:
- The basic equipment required for viewing the images and quality assurance testing
- Picture archiving and communication systems
- Storage and retrieval of images

INTRODUCTION

Breast services have become increasingly dependent on computers and digital technologies; working in conjunction with multiple electronic hospital data systems to give more accessible and transferrable patient records. Digital imaging is now the method by which mammography images are recorded and reviewed and usually works alongside the radiology information system (RIS) and, for breast screening in the United Kingdom, the national breast screening services (NBSS) computer system. A picture archiving and communication system (PACS) is the technology used to improve workflow, store, view, and share electronic images. The x-ray system can send the mammography images directly or indirectly to the PACS system, if, for example, the mobile unit is not networked. Each manufacturer has its own set of electronic instructions that ensure the images can be retrieved and viewed. PACS systems have a range of electronic functions enabling the user to manipulate the images, which can be used to enhance the image.

PICTURE ARCHIVING AND COMMUNICATION SYSTEMS

Hospital PACS systems provide a secured network for the transmission of mammography images in an electronic format. The patient demographics are received on the modality via a Digital Imaging Communication in Medicine (DICOM) Modality Worklist from the RIS. This provides all Key identifiers for patient examinations, images are sent from the mammography unit to PACS data store. The images are retrieved and reviewed on a dedicated workstation. The functionality and software applications will vary between manufacturers, but all will assist in diagnosis or exclusion of breast disease. Images may be sent electronically between hospitals, allowing transfer of patient records when they move or if a consultation between experts is needed. PACS is connected to RIS, which receives patient data updates from the hospital information system (HIS) or electronic patient record (EPR), this is connected to the patient summary care record (e.g., National Health Service [NHS] Spine), which is the primary patient data source. Updates from the HIS will cascade down through RIS to PACS to maintain patient data integrity (Fig. 2.1).

Acquisition Workstation

The acquisition workstation (AWS) is connected to the x-ray unit (Fig. 2.2) and allows the operator to view the images as soon as they are captured. A standard mammography acquisition monitor is 1 megapixel on a mobile unit but may be 3 megapixel in a static unit when linked to a stereotactic attachment.

Reporting Workstations

A diagnostic standard breast reporting workstation is used for making a primary diagnosis in breast disease. In screening, the monitor should allow the evaluation of two images at full size in full resolution, and it is recommended that diagnostic workstations have two matched 45 to 50 cm diagonal high quality 5 megapixel monitors. A breast reporting workstation usually comprises two reporting monitors and a third standard computer screen (Fig. 2.3). Workstations allow the reader to review a series of images in an entire sequence. The

Data flow is unidirectional

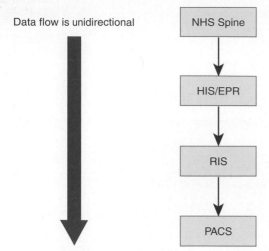

Fig. 2.1 Electronic data flow for digital images. *EPR*, Electronic patient record; *HIS*, hospital information system; *NHS*, National Health Service; *PACS*, picture archiving and communication system; *RIS*, radiology information system.

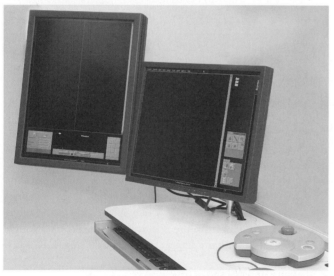

Fig. 2.2 Acquisition workstation.

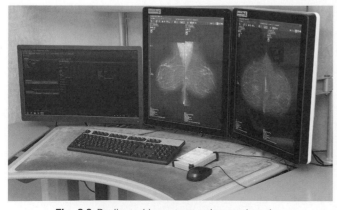

Fig. 2.3 Dedicated breast reporting workstation.

order in which the images are displayed is known as a hanging profile and may be adapted to the individual reader. Images must be retrievable for review or comparison with new examinations. There must be the ability to compare prior images, have correct orientation and annotation, adjustable contrast and gray scale, and images not obscured by annotation.

The image is sent to PACS, which triggers the prefetch function to retrieve relevant data and images from the historical examinations and attaches them to the patient folder for review, this is forwarded to the workstation.

If the network used is a local area network, the integration is with PACS. If a wide area network is used, the integration is with teleradiography.

After the image is available from the imaging system, the DICOM standard should be used for system integration. Image processing is performed to enhance visual quality. For example, in mammography, preprocessing functions include the segmentation of the breast from the background and the determination of the ranges of pixel value of various breast tissues for automatic window and level adjustment.

Systems Networks

A basic function of a computer system's network is to provide an access path by which end users at one geographic location can access information from another location. The infrastructure design will be determined by the purpose and use of the system, and consideration should be given to how information is transferred from remote mobile units.

Process coordination between tasks running on different computers connected to the network is an extremely important issue in systems networking.

PICTURE ARCHIVING AND COMMUNICATION SYSTEM INFRASTRUCTURE DESIGN

The four major factors in the PACS infrastructure design concepts are:
- System standardization
- Open architecture and connectivity
- Reliability
- Security

System Standardization

Adherence to industry standards and regulations for hardware and software makes the system easier to manage. Creating a standardized system following a clear set of rules will make the system more efficient and user friendly.

Open Architecture and Connectivity

All parts of the PACS system needs to be able to communicate in an integrated fashion with the system as a whole. If PACS modules in the same area cannot communicate with each other, potential problems arise as it is difficult to form a total integrated PACS if parts work independently. An open system allows for easier upgrade and system improvements.

Reliability

Because of the complexity and number of components associated with a PACS systems, the probability of failure is high and strong failsafe systems are essential.

Security

PACS systems hold a large amount of personal data, and patient confidentiality is a major consideration. Workstations should be in secure areas with locked doors and users logged off when not in use. There should be limited access to the systems (password and privilege controls) and staff awareness of data regulations.

IMAGE REVIEW

A standard four-view screening mammogram produces around 160 Mbytes of imaging data. These need to be retrieved and loaded to the workstation, ready for review in only a few seconds. The dedicated workstation has a number of functions that enable the reader to optimize the visualization of all of the breast tissue:

- Zoom and scroll can be used to magnify the image and move the image around the screen to focus on a region of interest.
- Window level feature allows the user to control the grouping and interval of gray levels to be displayed on the monitor.
- Image reverse can be used to reverse the dark and light pixels of an image.
- Distance calibration can be used to measure lesions and their position in the breast

TOMOSYNTHESIS

The review of tomosynthesis images requires adapted monitors (including quick refresh rate) suitable for tomosynthesis. A four-view mammogram obtained by tomosynthesis requires up to 1 GB of storage space and will use other viewing functions allowing image manipulation.

TESTING THE MONITORS

The monitors used for reporting should be tested daily. A digitally generated pattern is used to check imperfections of the display unit. The most commonly used digital phantom is the Society of Motion Picture and Television Engineers pattern (Fig. 2.4).

FURTHER READING

Carter, C. (2007). *Digital radiography and PACS.* London: Mosby.

Conant, E.F. (2014). Clinical implementation of digital breast tomosynthesis. *Radiologic Clinics of North America,* 52(3), 499–518.

European guidelines for quality assurance in breast cancer screening and diagnosis. Fourth edition. (2006). Luxembourg: Office for Official Publications of the European Communities.

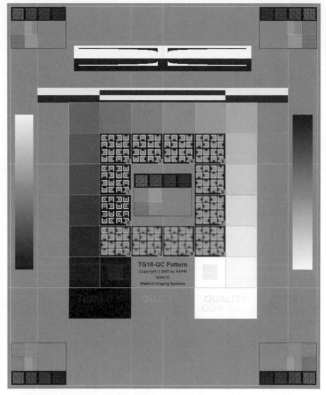

Fig. 2.4 Image quality test for breast reporting monitors.

Governance of radiology picture archiving and communication systems (PACS) following the United Kingdom deployment 2006-2010. (2011). The Royal college of Radiologists.

Guidelines and standards for implementation of new PACS/RIS solutions in the UK. (2011). The Royal College of radiologists.

Hogg, P., Kelly, J., Mercer, C. eds. (2015). *Digital mammography. A holistic approach.* Switzerland: Springer International Publishing.

Huang, H.K. (2010). *PACS and imaging informatics: basic principles and applications,* second edition. Wiley-Blackwell.

IAEA. (2016). *Digital Mammography Unit and Associated Services, Project GE06010.* Available at: https://www-pub.iaea.org/MTCD/Publications/PDF/Pub1482_web.pdf (Accessed 17/04/20).

Kanal, K.M., Krupinski, E., Berns, E.A., et al. (2013). ACR-AAPM-SIIM practice guideline for determinants of image quality in digital mammography. *Journal of Digital Imaging* 26(1), 10–25.

Kopans, D.B. (2006). *Breast imaging* (3rd ed). Baltimore, Maryland: Lippincott Williams & Wilkins.

NHS Cancer Screening Programmes. (2009). *Commissioning and Routine Testing of Full Field Digital Mammography Systems, Equipment Report 0604, Version 3.* Available at: https://assets.publishing.service.gov.uk/government/uploads/system/uploads/attachment_data/file/441857/nhsbsp-equipment-report-0604.pdf (Accessed 16/04/20).

Peck, A. (2017). Clark's essential PACS, RIS and imaging informatics. In *Clark's essential PACS, RIS and imaging informatics* (1st ed). CRC Press. Available at: https://doi.org/10.1201/9781315119823 accessed (Accessed 28/07/19).

Public Health England. (2019). *Breast screening: guidelines for medical physics services.* Breast Screening: Quality Assurance for Medical Physics Services. Available at: https://www.gov.uk/government/publications/breast-screening-quality-assurance-for-medical-physics-services/breast-screening-guidelines-for-medical-physics-services (Accessed 16/04/20).

Breast Anatomy: Implications for Mammographic Practice

OBJECTIVES

This chapter outlines:
- The embryology of the breast
- Normal breast development and activity
- Mammographic involution
- Interruptions to the involutionary process

- The anatomy of the adult breast
- Commonly encountered congenital anomalies
- The development of breast cancer
- Anatomically derived mammographic principles

EMBRYOLOGY

In humans, milk lines form as thickenings of the mammary ridge (Fig. 3.1), along the front surface of both male and female bodies. They appear in the seventh week of embryonic development before human sexual differentiation, which explains why male humans have nipples. Most of the tissue forming the ridges atrophies and disappears during embryonic life, leaving a single island on each side of the chest. Each of these develops into a rudimentary breast which persists throughout infancy and childhood. Occasionally, other islands of breast tissue persist at other sites along the ridges persisting as a separate accessory breast, or more commonly, an accessory nipple or simply a mole-like abnormality on the skin.

NORMAL DEVELOPMENT

Glandular Tissue

About 15 to 20 rods of tissue grow down from the apex of the island of lactogenic tissue into the rudimentary tissue beneath. The rods branch successively as they penetrate deeply and ultimately become hollow. These are the breast ducts. The terminal portions of the branching system are where the functioning breast tissues form. The terminal ducts branch into ductules from which buds grow. These buds open out to form lobules, the epithelial-lined cavities, which are the milk-producing glandular elements of the breast. A terminal duct and the associated lobules arising from it are called the terminal ductolobular unit (TDLU). These TDLUs are the most important part of the breast, from the point of view of both normal physiologic function and the development of breast disease. Not only do most benign conditions have their origin in this area, but it is from the epithelial cells lining the TDLUs that breast cancers arise.

Postnatal Development

In females, the hormonal influences of puberty cause further development of the rudimentary breast tissues. Increased branching of the duct system leads to an increase in the number of TDLUs. The TDLUs themselves increase in size by proliferation in the number and size of the epithelial cells lining each lobular cavity and by expansion of the ductal and lobular lamina. Approximately 20% of adolescent boys also experience some degree of breast development (gynecomastia), which is usually transient.

On a mammogram, each TDLU casts a shadow about 1 mm in diameter. When development is complete, at around the age of 20 years, there are many hundreds of TDLUs completely filling the breast. Superimposition of the TDLU shadows forms the uniform overall density of the breast seen on mammography.

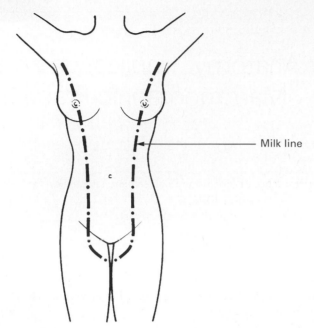

Fig. 3.1 The milk line, running from clavicle to groin.

The breast is divided into 15 to 20 segments or lobes. Each segment contains a network of ducts that drain the TDLUs. Under the nipple, these ducts coalesce to form lactiferous sinuses which, in turn, drain out through the nipple. In the breast, there are fibrous septa (ligaments of Astley Cooper) that divide and support the segments. There are two types of tissues within each segment: glandular tissue, supported in a stroma of fibrofatty tissue (Fig. 3.2).

Accessory Breast Tissue

It is not uncommon for the islands of glandular tissue developing in the lactogenic ridges to grow in two parts, with an additional small collection immediately adjacent to the main island of tissue, usually above but sometimes below. Although the development of accessory breast tissue is usually bilateral, it is not always symmetrical, and may be unilateral. The accessory breast tissue can be visualized on a mammogram as a separate island of normal-looking glandular tissue lying within the breast (Fig. 3.3A and B). The condition may be noticed as a palpable mass by a woman or her clinician, but the anxiety generated by this discovery is readily relieved on inspection of the mammogram.

NORMAL ACTIVITY

From maturity to menopause with interruptions for pregnancy, there are associated with each menstrual cycle, alternating increases and decreases in the size and activity of the epithelial cells lining each TDLU.

The cyclic increases and decreases are not usually associated with any perceptible change in mammographic appearance. It may, however, be difficult for a mammographer to obtain adequate compression if a breast is tender during the premenstrual phase. In this situation, a mammogram may be

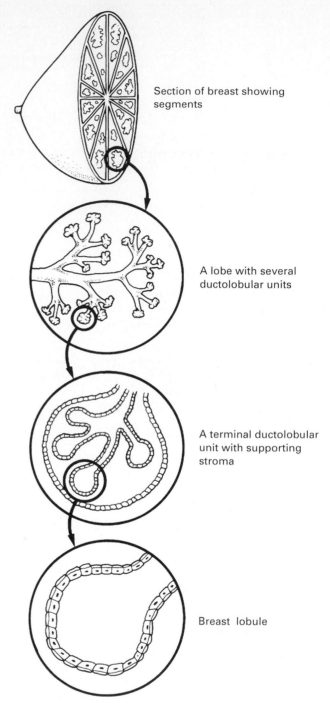

Fig. 3.2 Diagram of breast tissue at progressively increasing magnifications.

of inferior quality and will therefore appear different, being more dense than one taken with proper compression. Should a mammographer encounter difficulties in examining a woman in the premenstrual part of her cycle, then the examination may be best deferred until mid-cycle. For the same reason, if a woman has suffered undue discomfort or pain during a mammographic examination in the past, future examinations are better scheduled to be undertaken in mid-cycle.

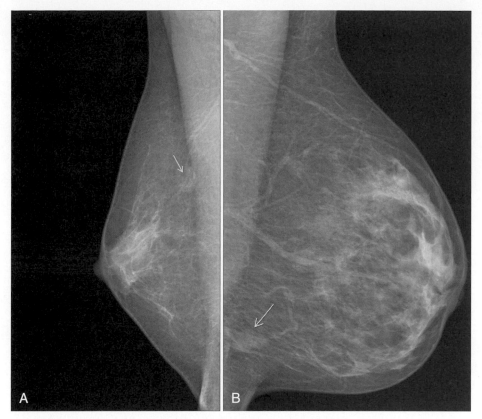

Fig. 3.3 Accessory breast tissue: (A) above the main breast; (B) below the main breast.

MAMMOGRAPHIC INVOLUTION

It is important not to confuse the mammographic appearance of a dense or fatty breast pattern with the process of physiologic involution. The density of the breast tissues on mammography depends upon a number of factors: the amount of glandular tissue, the amount of fibrous tissue, and the degree of obesity of the woman. In general, younger women will have dense breast tissue, while older women will have fatty breast tissue, however some 20% of women at age 30 years have a fatty appearance, and approximately 40% of 80-year-olds have a dense pattern (Fig. 3.4).

Physiologic involution of the breast glandular tissue starts virtually as soon as a woman is mature and can be regarded as the reverse of development. The TDLUs decrease in size, eventually being replaced by fibrous tissue and fat. This process is quite different from the concept of mammographic involution.

Mammographic involution is the process of progressive reduction in the density of breast tissue. This is associated with a reduction in the proportion of the breast which is occupied by that density and also the change in shape of the dense portion. This process may be obscured completely in a breast with a high fibrous tissue content.

Evidence of mammographic involution is seen initially in the periphery of the breast, noted on a mammogram as an increase in the size of the layer of fat in the subcutaneous and

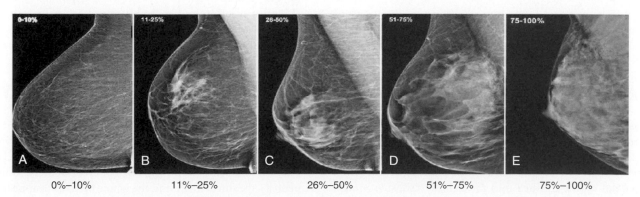

| 0%–10% | 11%–25% | 26%–50% | 51%–75% | 75%–100% |

Fig. 3.4 Increasing background breast density from almost entirely fatty to very dense.

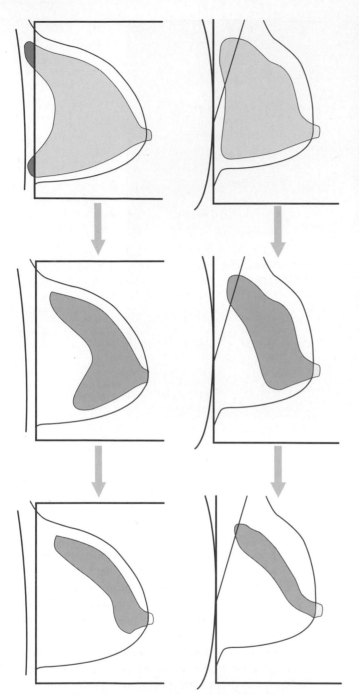

Fig. 3.5 Process of mammographic involution.

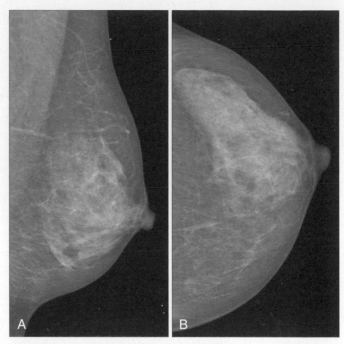

Fig. 3.6 Mammograms of partially involuted breast showing oblique orientation of uninvoluted tissue (A) MLO; (B) CC.

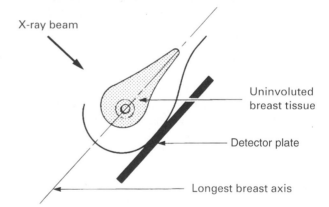

Fig. 3.7 The MLO illustrating maximal demonstration of breast tissue without foreshortening.

retromammary regions. The breast tissue densities then start to shrink and finally disappear. The tissues in the lower inner quadrant change more rapidly than those in the upper inner and lower outer quadrants, with those in the superolateral quadrant usually the last to show change (Fig. 3.5). By the time the woman reaches the age when a routine mammography is indicated, mammographic involution of the breast is reasonably well advanced, particularly inferiorly and medially. The residual visible uninvoluted disc of glandular tissue density is then orientated in an oblique plane extending from behind the nipple upward into the axillary tail, surrounded by a layer of fatty tissue (Fig. 3.6). In view of the orientation of the glandular breast tissue, the mediolateral oblique (MLO) projection, rather than a lateral, is vitally important to ensure as much breast tissue is visualised as possible without foreshortening (Fig. 3.7). The advantages of this projection are now universally accepted.

INTERRUPTIONS TO THE INVOLUTIONARY PROCESS

Pregnancy

With pregnancy, each TDLU hypertrophies to become larger than the size achieved during normal cyclic activity. Simultaneously, the ducts dilate and the whole breast will appear very dense on a mammogram. Mammography should only be performed in exceptional circumstances during pregnancy. Following the cessation of lactation, the breast reverts to the prepregnancy appearance within a few weeks. Thereafter, the slow disappearance of glandular density continues at the same rate as before the pregnancy.

Hormone Replacement Therapy

The use of hormone replacement therapy (HRT) can impact on the mammographic density of the breast. Effectively it represses, and to some degree reverses, the mammographic involutionary process. The impact of HRT on breast pattern varies dependent on the individual, and the type or length of usage of HRT. However, studies to date have shown that the increase in breast density increases the recall rate in a breast screening service and this may have implications for the future if the use of HRT continues to rise.

Influence of Hormone Replacement Therapy on Breast Cancer Risk

With the increase in HRT use, concern has been expressed that women using HRT may be at increased risk of developing breast cancer. The baseline risk of breast cancer for women around menopausal age varies from one woman to another according to the presence of underlying risk factors. HRT with estrogen alone is associated with little or no change in the risk of breast cancer. HRT with estrogen and progestogen can be associated with an increase in the risk of breast cancer. Any increase in the risk of breast cancer is related to treatment duration and reduces after stopping HRT.

ANATOMY OF THE ADULT FEMALE BREAST

The external form of the adult female breast varies enormously, but its attachment to the chest wall is constant, extending from the fourth to the sixth ribs vertically and from the costal cartilage to the anterior axillary fold transversely. The upper outer quadrant includes a prolongation of breast tissue, known as the axillary tail, which extends toward the axilla. The external rounded form of the breast does not represent the shape of the glandular tissue within the breast. The shape of the breast is caused by the fatty tissue which surrounds the glandular elements and which replaces glandular tissue as involution progresses with age.

CONGENITAL ANOMALIES

A congenital anomaly occurs when the normal sequence of developmental events takes place in a disordered fashion. Most of the breast anomalies are of academic interest only, but there are a few that are important to a mammographer.

Post- and Prefixed Breasts

In the adult female, the developed breast is an approximately hemispherical disc attached by its base to the anterior chest

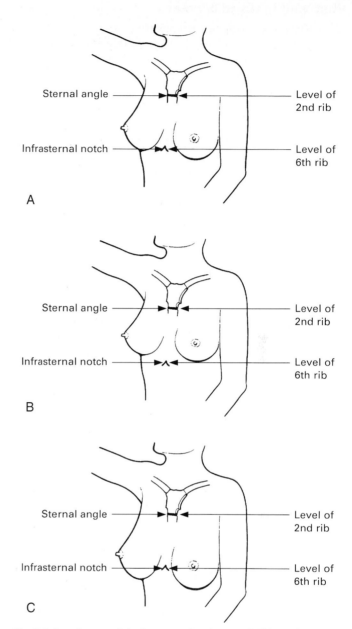

Fig. 3.8 Attachment of the breast to the chest wall: (A) usual position (2nd to 6th rib); (B) prefixed; (C) postfixed.

wall and extends from the fourth rib above to the sixth rib below (Fig. 3.8A). Occasionally, the main island of breast tissue happens, by chance, to develop in a position higher (prefixed) or lower (postfixed) than is usual (Fig. 3.8B and C). In either case, the relationship of the breast to the underlying pectoralis muscle will be abnormal, and this will be obvious on an MLO mammogram. In a woman with a prefixed breast, the upper border of the breast can lie as high as the second rib, when its close proximity to the clavicle can make it difficult to achieve satisfactory positioning for adequate mammography. In women with postfixed breasts, the ribs lying above the breast are often clearly evident and the detector plate will need to be placed at a lower level than the norm.

Post- and Prefixed Nipples

A breast may be in the normal position on the chest wall, but the nipple and areola may develop in an unusually high or low position. Again, this will be obvious on viewing a MLO mammogram, when there will be an altered relationship between the nipple and the lower corner of the pectoralis shadow. It can be difficult to project pre- and postfixed nipples in profile, particularly in the craniocaudal position, and it may be necessary to take a special nipple view.

BREAST CANCER DEVELOPMENT

Breast cancer arises from the epithelial lining of the ducts and lobules. The triggers that create the right environment for the onset of the disease process are not yet fully established, but these triggers cause the cells to behave in an aberrant way. Normal cells have a finite life and are replaced by newly developed cells on a regular basis. This is the normal process for cells throughout the body. With breast cancer, the cells do not die but continue to thrive and multiply within the confines of the ductal space. Although confined to the ductal system, the disease, although present, cannot spread and is known as in situ disease.

Once the cancer cells have broken through the basement membrane of the ductal system, there is potential for a spread into the surrounding breast tissue, the vascular and lymphatic systems, and potentially to the rest of the body. Histopathologists apply terms, such as minimally invasive or microinvasive to indicate early stages of invasion into the surrounding tissue. Broadly speaking, the smaller the invasive component, the less likelihood of spread. However, this depends on a multiplicity of factors which lie beyond the remit of this book.

As indicated in subsequent chapters, early stages of breast cancer development can be identified in the majority of cases with mammography. Given some basic understanding of breast cancer development, a mammographer will be fully aware of the potential benefits of mammography to the diagnostic process.

ANATOMICALLY DERIVED MAMMOGRAPHIC PRINCIPLES

- The object of mammography is to demonstrate breast glandular tissue, not fatty tissue or skin. In all projections, it is the internal glandular tissue which should be considered and not the outer form of the breast.
- Normal variations on gross anatomy of the breast will influence mammographic technique (see Ch. 7).
- It is a fundamental principle of radiography that the x-ray beam is directed at right angles to the longest diameter of the body part to be imaged to avoid foreshortening. Because it is not the breast fat but the glandular tissue which has to be demonstrated on a mammogram, the longest diameter is that which extends into the upper outer quadrant, at about 45 degrees to the horizontal. It follows that, apart from the MLO, all projections cause foreshortening of the uninvoluted gland tissue.

- In all projections, the breast should be lifted so that the nipple is level with the center of the circular attachment of the breast to the chest wall, that is, to the level of the fourth rib.
- For the MLO projection, the detector plate angle should be adjusted to reflect the particular stature of the woman (Fig. 3.7). Varying the angle, to suit the stature of the woman, will ensure that the beam is at right angles to the longest diameter of the glandular tissue, minimizing foreshortening compression and will be parallel to the correctly positioned pectoralis major, thus reducing the woman's discomfort. Approximate angles from the horizontal are as follows:
  i. 40 degrees for a short, stocky woman
  ii. 45 degrees for the average woman
  iii. 50 degrees for a tall woman of slim build.
- Because the breast is attached to a curved chest wall, it is inevitable that some breast tissue will be "cut off" and not be demonstrated on the film (see Chs. 5 and 6). Knowledge of breast development and involutionary processes ensure that any areas excluded will contain fat rather than glandular tissue.
- The comparative mobility of the lateral portions of the breast compared with the medial should be factors considered in mammographic positioning.

FURTHER READING

Andolina, V. (2011). *Mammographic imaging: a practical guide* (3rd ed.). Philadelphia: Wolters Kluwer/Lippincott Williams & Wilkins Health.

Azam S., Lange T., Huynh S., et al. (2018). Hormone replacement therapy, mammographic density, and breast cancer risk: a cohort study. *Cancer Causes & Control*, 29, 495–505.

Bland, K.I., Copeland, E.M., Klimberg, V.S., Gradishar, W.J. (2017). The breast: comprehensive management of benign and malignant diseases. In *The breast: comprehensive management of benign and malignant diseases*. Elsevier Inc.

Dixon, J.M. (ed). (2012). *ABC of breast diseases* 4th Edition. London, BMJ Books.

Dumky, H., Leifland, K., Fridell, K. (2018). The art of mammography with respect to positioning and compression—a Swedish perspective. *Journal of Radiology Nursing*, 37(1), 41–48.

Feng, Y., Spezia, M., Huang, S., et al. (2018). Breast cancer development and progression: risk factors, cancer stem cells, signaling pathways, genomics, and molecular pathogenesis. *Genes and Diseases*, 5, 2, 77–106.

Hogg, P., Kelly, J., Mercer, C. (2015). *Digital mammography*. Springer International Publishing.

Jatoi, I., Kaufmann, M. (2016). *Management of breast diseases*. Springer International Publishing.

Javed, A., Lteif, A. (2013). Development of the human breast. *Seminars in Plastic Surgery*, 27(1), 5–12.

Kopans, D.B. (2006). *Breast imaging* (3rd ed). Baltimore, Maryland: Lippincott Williams & Wilkins.

Popli, M.B., Teotia, R., Narang, M., Krishna, H. (2014). Breast positioning during mammography: mistakes to be avoided. *Breast Cancer: Basic and Clinical Research*, 20144:8, 119–124.

Prebil, L.A., Ereman, R.R., Powell, M.J., et al. (2014). First pregnancy events and future breast density: modification by age at first pregnancy and specific VEGF and IGF1R gene variants. *Cancer Causes & Control*, 25, 859–868.

Schoenwolf, G.C., Bleyl, S.B., Brauer, P.R., Francis-West, P.H. (2015) (eds). *Larsen's human embryology*, 5th Edition. Philadelphia: Churchill Livingstone.

Shetty, M.K. ed. (2014). *Breast cancer screening and diagnosis: a synopsis*. New York: Springer.

Shiffman, M. (2009). Breast Augmentation. In M. A. Shiffman (Ed.), *Breast augmentation: principles and practice* 1st ed. (pp. 1–672). Berlin Heidelberg: Springer.

Skandalakis, J.E. (2009). 'Embryology and anatomy of the breast'. In M.A., Shiffman (ed), *Breast augmentation: principles and practice* (pp 3–24). Berlin Heidelberg: Springer.

Mammography: The First Steps

OBJECTIVES

This chapter outlines:
- Importance of clinical background
- Issues of consent and justification of radiation exposure
- Communication and the development of a rapport with the women

- Points of technique relating to all examinations, including anatomic positioning—the "whole body" technique
- Compression of the breast—why and how

UNDERSTANDING THE CLINICAL BACKGROUND

Every woman who attends for mammography deserves to be treated as an individual. Women attend a mammography unit for a variety of reasons:
- National or local screening programs
- Family history surveillance
- Breast symptoms
- Additional views
- Stereotactic-guided needle biopsy and/or localization procedures
- Research studies
- Follow-up mammography

If the woman has been referred for a mammogram because of symptoms, rather than for breast cancer screening, she is more likely to be well motivated to attend. It is likely that she will be tolerant of the procedure and may openly express her anxieties regarding the outcome. Among these, she may already have faced the possibility that her symptoms could be caused by cancer. It is more likely that a woman with symptoms will take the opportunity to discuss her problems and anxieties with a mammographer than will a woman attending for screening. The mammographer should be aware of this, and be prepared to accept the role of sympathetic listener.

In contrast, a woman attending for screening is normally well and without symptoms, and her expectations are likely to differ from those presenting with a problem. She could be resentful of the procedure and is likely to expect a higher degree of efficiency, such as keeping to appointment times. She may be more anxious about the procedure and less likely to tolerate discomfort. The possible dangers of radiation may be worrying her, and she may be fearful of the results. Women attending for screening usually expect a normal outcome, while those with symptoms are likely to be better prepared for an abnormal result.

Knowing the reason for the attendance can help the mammographer in assessing the woman's likely psychological state in relation to the examination. As well as providing essential information, the clinical background will assist in establishing rapport and the validity of the imaging request.

Records of previous attendances will give an insight into particular difficulties or the need for variation of technique. Previous mammograms are of value so that an assessment can be made of unusual mammographic appearances requiring additional projections or a variation in exposure technique. Previous mammograms and correctly completed imaging requests can also give an indication of a woman's previous clinical history.

JUSTIFYING THE EXPOSURE

All medical doses of ionizing radiation are governed by stringent regulation. The mammographer who administers the radiation exposure; known as an operator in the Ionizing Radiation (Medical Exposure) Regulations (IR[ME]R)—must be certain that the appropriate justification for administering the dose has been provided. If the examination request does not provide sufficient clinical information, the mammographer should ask the referrer for clarification.

Departments should have protocols and standard operating procedures clarifying acceptable practice under most circumstances. If a request goes outside the normal protocols and the woman may be at risk from unnecessary radiation, the mammographer should not proceed until the request is justified. A good knowledge and understanding of imaging protocols and, more importantly, the rationale behind them will help the mammographer make the correct, professional decision thus providing the best care for the woman. Trainees, assistant practitioners, and associate mammographers/apprentices will need to refer to the appropriate professional for further advice under some circumstances, as it may be outside of their scope of practice for them to proceed with some investigations.

ISSUES OF INFORMED OR VALID CONSENT

It is not the purpose of this book to set out the legal debate on consent because of the widespread variability. However, every professional should ensure that they have an understanding of these issues and the local approach to this. It is essential that the mammographer is sure that the woman attending has enough knowledge on which to proceed with the examination or decline if she so wishes.

Women invited to breast screening are issued an information leaflet alongside their appointment letter detailing risks and benefits of the breast screening program so that when they attend their appointment, informed consent is implied. This can be clarified on attendance by the mammographer.

Women with symptoms may have different concerns and anxieties to those with no symptoms, requiring different information and communication techniques, but in all cases, the mammographer needs to recognize when the woman who has arrived willingly, has the capacity to give consent, and/or later withdraws consent at some point during the procedure.

A complication of informed consent relates to those who are brought to the unit by relatives or professional care staff, and those who may have physical, emotional, or mental challenges. Breast screening should be available to all eligible women, and women in these groups can be assisted to understand the process and appropriate adaptations made to meet the individual needs. It should be noted that the individual has the final choice and the mammographer needs to be sensitive to their wishes, however these are demonstrated.

An important part of consent is the limitations of mammography. Women who present with a symptomatic breast cancer between screening appointments, or women representing symptomatically after a short time interval, may ask probing questions about their previous mammograms. Women have the right to know the outcome of any audit review of their previous investigations that may have resulted in a cancer being misinterpreted or misdiagnosed.

PREMAMMOGRAPHY DISCUSSION

Establishing Rapport

Good communication skills are essential to successful mammography investigations. A woman's perception of a mammographic service largely depends on the performance and communication skills of the mammographer. It takes great skill to balance a relaxed woman and a timely completion of the mammogram investigation. There is limited opportunity for the mammographer to communicate with a woman within the short appointment times. A woman's anxiety will be significantly increased if insufficient time is available for her and the mammographer to communicate.

The best opportunity to build up a rapport with a woman is immediately before the examination. This is necessary to help her feel comfortable about the examination. Having a physically relaxed woman is an essential prerequisite to obtaining high-quality mammography. Any question the woman raises should be answered frankly and openly. If a mammographer does not know the answer, they should say so and suggest a likely source for information. It is important the mammographer should not give reassurance beyond their own field of competence. In the technological age, women have easy access to information through the internet and social media, although not all of this information will be reliable in nature, it may influence the type of questions raised.

Explaining the Procedure

Time should be spent with the woman explaining the examination. A woman attending for the first time may have heard an inaccurate account of the mammographic examination from numerous potential sources. The information they have about mammography may be wildly inaccurate, resulting in increased anxiety levels. To obtain maximum cooperation, these fears should be countered with a clear concise explanation of exactly what the examination entails. Phrases to use during the explanation might include comments such as:

- "It is uncomfortable rather than painful."
- "If it does become too uncomfortable, don't hesitate to tell me."
- "It doesn't last long—only a few seconds for each image."
- "Compression is essential to obtain good pictures and to show details clearly."
- "The pressure will not harm your breasts."

Relevant History

In many screening units, it is the usual practice for the mammographer to take a brief medical history before the examination. This is useful both in establishing rapport and in obtaining information about relevant breast symptoms, which could assist in the later interpretation of the mammograms by the reader. However, any symptomatic imaging request should contain all the necessary information to facilitate the correct interpretation of any images. Details worth recording include:

- A brief summary of the reason for the current examination
- Past history of breast disease, the suspected diagnosis at the time, and any treatment given, especially the site and date of any previous surgery

- Details of any scars or skin lesions should be marked on a diagram
- Any reported breast symptom
- Some centers feel it is appropriate to record any history of breast cancer in the family
- In some centers, a note is also made of any hormone replacement therapy, including duration and type of treatment.

Observing and Reporting Clinical Signs

All women attending for symptomatic clinics will have perceived symptoms; however, some women attending for screening will also report symptoms. It is important to note relevant symptoms and the woman's concerns for those reading the images. It is also important for the mammographer to note details of any significant clinical signs they may observe during the procedure. Local protocols will outline relevant signs and symptoms which are important. The NHSBSP also provides guidance for mammographers, these signs may indicate an underlying abnormality which may not be demonstrated on mammography and could bring to the attention of the team an occult breast cancer. Important signs to note include:

- A new lump
- Skin tethering or dimpling
- Recent nipple inversion
- Eczema of the nipple
- Nipple discharge

It is recommended that mammographers spend some time in a breast clinic with a specialist clinician, observing the examination of women with symptoms so that skills in recognizing significant clinical signs of breast disease are acquired.

IMPORTANT POINTS OF TECHNIQUE

There are some points of technique that apply to all mammographic projections and that should be regarded as "golden rules." The following notes outline the more important of these.

Image Annotation

Care should be taken to check the identity of the woman, and to make sure that the correct woman is selected from the work list. Annotation and anatomic legends will be electronically applied according to the imaging protocol selected. The mammographer must follow the order of the protocol they have selected, as the system will orientate the digital images to match the selected protocol. Any deviation will need to be selected manually for the annotation to be corrected. The mammographer must ensure all information is correct before forwarding any image to the picture archiving and communication system (PACS). Most units will have a minimum dataset required to uniquely identify any given woman.

Anatomic Positioning

From the point of view of positioning, mammography is a whole-body technique. The correct positioning of the woman's feet, arms, and spine are important in obtaining high-quality diagnostic mammograms. It is essential therefore to consider all these aspects of positioning throughout the examination. The position of the woman's whole body must be manipulated and controlled by the mammographer for the breast to be examined properly. This task is most easily achieved by performing the examination with the woman standing.

On occasions, a woman may have to be examined while she is seated, and it is perfectly possible to achieve excellent mammograms in this position. Specially designed examination chairs with full and adjustable lumbar support make this task much simpler for the woman and the examining mammographer. The chair should be on wheels, with an easily operated, foot-activated braking system.

Manipulating and Controlling the Breast

Handling the breast can be difficult for the mammographer, particularly in early stages of training. The mammographer should be firm but considerate, the hand cupping of the breast with the thumb and fingers at the posterior margin of the breast against the chest wall; the internal structures of the breast must be maneuvered into the correct position, not just the overlying fat. Control of the breast throughout the procedure is essential to high-quality images. Mammography is a very intimate examination with some level of discomfort for many women, consideration to her needs and her experience during every investigation will influence both the quality of the resultant images and the likelihood of her continuing to attend for breast screening in the future.

COMPRESSION OF THE BREAST

Compression of the breast tissue is essential for good mammography. Before an examination, the woman should be clearly and simply told about the need for breast compression. It is then more likely that she will tolerate the examination. Beneficial effects of breast compression during mammography include:

- Reduction of internal x-ray beam scatter
- Improved contrast
- Spreading of breast tissues:
  - reduced superimposition
  - clearer demonstration
- Reduced geometric unsharpness
- Reduced movement unsharpness
- Reduced radiation dose to the breast
- More homogeneous film density

When applying compression, control of the whole woman should be maintained, as detailed earlier, with one hand guiding the position of the woman's body, while the other manipulates the breast. As the compression paddle descends onto the breast and begins to hold it firmly, the hand controlling the breast should be moved forward slowly from the chest wall toward the nipple. Care should be taken to ensure that the hand does not itself take any of the compression force. There is considerable skill involved in applying compression without losing control of the breast position; the novice will almost certainly experience some difficulties with this initially.

Selection of the correct compression paddle will improve the ability to apply the correct compression to the breast. This will also ensure correct exposure factors are applied and the subsequent images are displayed correctly on the PACS workstations.

There is an optimum level of compression beyond which extra force ceases to have any perceptible effect on image quality or any significant reduction in radiation dose. However, the additional force does have a marked effect on the woman's tolerance of the procedure. "Discomfort" becomes "pain" if that "little bit more" compression is applied. This may then cause the woman to decline further invitations for breast screening in the future.

In the United Kingdom, the maximum force permitted to be applied to the breast is 200 newtons (N). The majority of recently produced machines have a limiting level of approximately 160 N. In normal practice, this amount of force should not be necessary.

FURTHER READING

Al-Shdaifat, E.A. (2015). Implementation of total quality management in hospitals. *Journal of Taibah University Medical Sciences*, 10(4), 461–466.

Andolina, V. (2011). *Mammographic imaging: a practical guide* (3rd ed.). Philadelphia: Wolters Kluwer/Lippincott Williams & Wilkins Health.

Dixon, J.M. (ed). (2012). *ABC of breast diseases 4th Edition*. London: BMJ Books.

Department of Health and Social Care. (2017). *Guidance to the Ionising Radiation (Medical Exposure) Regulations 2017*. gov.uk. Available at: https://www.gov.uk/government/publications/ionising-radiation-medical-exposure-regulations-2017-guidance (Accessed 3/1/2020).

Dumky, H., Leifland, K., Fridell, K. (2018). The art of mammography with respect to positioning and compression—A Swedish perspective. *Journal of Radiology Nursing*, 37(1), 41–48.

Guertin, M.H., Théberge, I., Dufresne, M.P., et al. (2014). Clinical image quality in daily practice of breast cancer mammography screening. *Canadian Association of Radiologists Journal*, 65(3), 199–206.

Hogg, P., Kelly, J., Mercer, C. (2015). *Digital mammography* (eds.). Springer International Publishing.

Jasper, M. (2013). *Beginning reflective practice* (2nd ed). Andover: Cengage Learning.

Kopans, D.B. (2006). *Breast imaging* (3rd ed). Baltimore, Maryland: Lippincott Williams & Wilkins.

Marmot, M.G., Altman, D.G., Cameron, A.D., Dewar, J.A., Thompson, S.G., Wilcox, M. (2013). The benefits and harms of breast cancer screening; an independent review. *British Journal of Cancer*, 108(11), 2205–2240.

Nightingale, J.M., Murphy, F.J., Robinson, L., Newton-Hughes, A., Hogg, P. (2015). Breast compression - An exploration of problem solving and decision-making in mammography. *Radiography*, 21(4), 364–369.

Perry, N., Broeders, M., de Wolf, C., Törnberg, S., Holland, R., von Karsa, L. (2008). European guidelines for quality assurance in breast cancer screening and diagnosis. —summary document. *Annals of Oncology*, 19(4), 614–622.

Public Health England. (2017b). NHS Breast Screening Programme Guidance for breast screening mammographers. 3rd Ed. Available at: https://assets.publishing.service.gov.uk/government/uploads/system/uploads/attachment_data/file/819410/NHS_Breast_Screening_Programme_Guidance_for_mammographers_final.pdf (Accessed 16/04/20).

Public Health England. (2018). Guidance: Interval cancers and applying duty of candour. Available at: https://www.gov.uk/government/publications/breast-screening-interval-cancers-and-duty-of-candour-toolkit/interval-cancers-and-applying-duty-of-candour (Accessed 19/03/20).

Public Health England. (2019). NHS breast screening: Helping you decide. https://assets.publishing.service.gov.uk/government/uploads/system/uploads/attachment_data/file/840343/Breast_screening_helping_you_decide.pdf (Accessed 19/03/20).

Rubin, C. (2019). *Guidance on screening and symptomatic breast imaging*. (4th Ed) https://www.rcr.ac.uk/system/files/publication/field_publication_files/bfcr199-guidance-on-screening-and-symptomatic-breast-imaging.pdf.

The Royal College of Radiologists. (2019). *Guidance on screening and symptomatic breast imaging 4th edition*. November. Clinical Radiology. Available at: https://www.rcr.ac.uk/system/files/publication/field_publication_files/bfcr199-guidance-on-screening-and-symptomatic-breast-imaging.pdf (Accessed 20/04/20).

Waade, G.G., SebuØdegård, S., Hogg, P., Hofvind, S. (2018). Breast compression across consecutive examinations among females participating in BreastScreen Norway. *British Journal of Radiology*, 91(1090), 20180209.

5

Mammography: Basic Projections

CHAPTER CONTENTS

OBJECTIVES

This chapter outlines:
- How to perform the basic mammographic projections: the craniocaudal and the mediolateral oblique

- How to recognize and rectify positioning faults as they arise
- How to recognize the adequacy of the examination

INTRODUCTION

Mammography is a highly technical examination. Producing consistent high quality mammograms on a range of women requires a skilled mammographer. This chapter describes a standard technique, but every examination is unique and will require the mammographer to make the examination acceptable to the woman with minimal loss of quality. Poor quality images can play a significant part in the misdiagnosis of breast disease. For each examination, the mammographer will need to make an ergonomic assessment of the woman to be examined in the context of her own physical capabilities and limitations.

The combination of the craniocaudal (CC) and the mediolateral oblique (MLO) mammograms are the routine projections for all initial x-ray examinations of the breast. This chapter aims to describe positioning for a high-quality mammogram demonstrating all of the breast tissue. This is not achievable on all women, and Chapter 9 explains how to critique the resultant images, to enable the mammographer to decide if her images are satisfactory or require repeating.

THE CRANIOCAUDAL PROJECTION

Area Demonstrated

The CC projection demonstrates the breast from top to bottom. The majority of breast tissue is demonstrated with the exclusion of the extreme medial portion and the axillary tail (Figs. 5.1 and 5.2).

Equipment Position

The detector plate is horizontal and raised to slightly above the level of inframammary angle.

Anatomic Position: Left Breast

The woman faces the machine, about 5 to 6 cm away, with her feet pointing toward the machine. Her arms are relaxed by her side and her head turned slightly to the right. The breast to be examined should be aligned with the center of the detector plate (Fig. 5.3). The mammographer should stand medial of the breast to be examined.

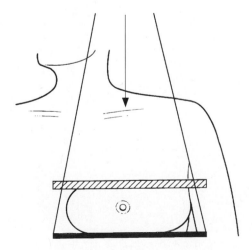

Fig. 5.1 The craniocaudal projection.

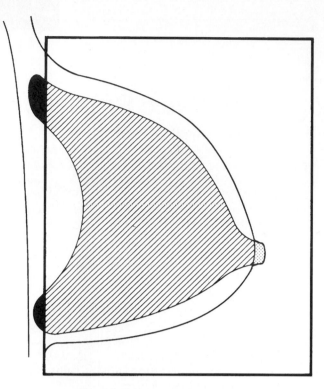

Fig. 5.2 The area demonstrated.

Breast Positioning

a. Ask the woman to lean in slightly and lift the left breast up and away from the chest wall with your right hand (Fig. 5.4).

b. Encourage her to relax her shoulder.

c. Keep her head turned to the right.

d. Check the tissue is pulled from the inframammary fold (Fig. 5.5).

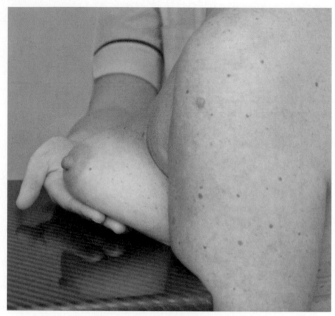

Fig. 5.4 Lift the breast up and away from the chest wall.

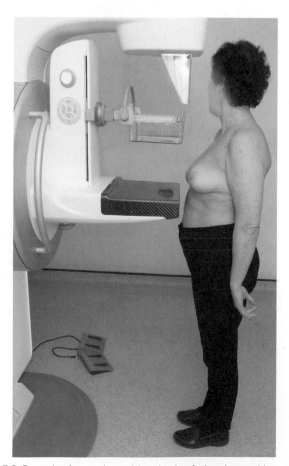

Fig. 5.3 Preparing for craniocaudal projection facing the machine, arms relaxed by the side.

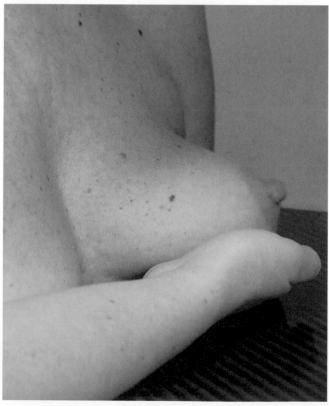

Fig. 5.5 Check the inframammary fold for creases.

e. Encourage her to keep leaning forward, with the thorax rotated a few degrees medially to bring the rib cage directly below the nipple line against the edge of the detector plate. The detector plate is close to the rib cage and inframammary angle, the nipple is forward and the whole breast supported (Fig. 5.6).

f. Maintaining the relaxed left shoulder, using both hands from beneath the breast, pull the glandular breast tissue forward and away from the rib cage onto the detector plate. This will ensure all of the glandular tissue is included on the resultant image (Fig. 5.7).

g. Ensure the breast is in the correct position, ready to apply optimum compression. Using the light beam diaphragm, check that the area to be demonstrated is included in the radiation field as shown in Fig. 5.2 including:
   i. the nipple in profile
   ii. the medial portion of the breast on the film
   iii. the shoulder is relaxed in order that the upper lateral portion of the breast on the film
   iv. the image field covers all the tissue in front of the thorax
   If the criteria are not achieved, refer to Table 5.1.

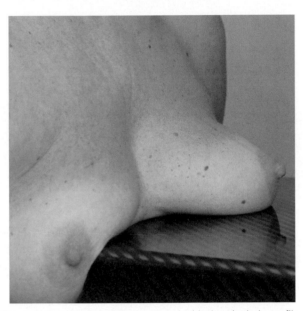

Fig. 5.6 The breast is fully supported with the nipple in profile.

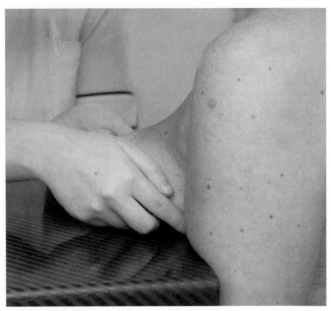

Fig. 5.7 Pull medial and lateral borders of the breast fully onto the detector plate.

TABLE 5.1	Trouble Shooting for Craniocaudal Projection	
Problem	**Cause**	**Corrective Action**
Nipple pointing downward	The detector plate is too high	Decrease the height of the detector plate
	The skin on the underside of the breast is caught at the edge of the detector plate	Lift the breast again, pulling forward the underside of the breast
	Excess loose skin on the superior surface of the breast	Control the nipple position by gently applying tension to the skin surface as compression is applied. Note: Move only the skin surface, not the underlying tissue
	The woman has a postfixed nipple	No improvement can be made without loss of breast tissue
		Either take a supplementary view and/or ensure a clear view of the retroareolar region on the mediolateral oblique
Folds at the lateral aspect	Pad of fat/skin above upper outer quadrant	Alter the position of the arm: a. Put her hand on her hip b. Put the palm of her hand on her abdomen c. Put her hand on her shoulder with her elbow back d. Bring her hand forward beneath support table to hold on at the far side
	The woman is leaning toward the medial	Lift the breast, encourage her to step a little to the medial and lean to the lateral
	The breast is twisted	Using the flat of your right hand, lift the breast and push the superior surface laterally, and pull the inferior surface medially

Applying the Compression

a. Maintaining a relaxed shoulder, using the palm of your right hand on the superior surface, pull gently forward toward the nipple, keeping the tissue pulled away from the rib cage (Fig. 5.8).

b. Using the foot pedal, apply compression slowly and evenly, keep the back of the breast pulled in by gradually moving your hand toward the nipple until the hand is replaced by the compression plate (Fig. 5.9).

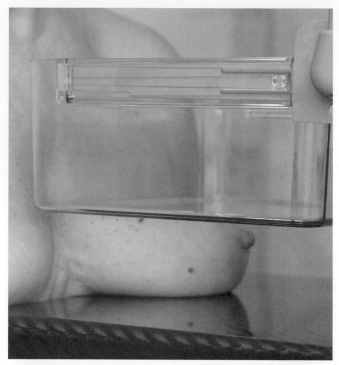

Fig. 5.10 Final position check before completing compression.

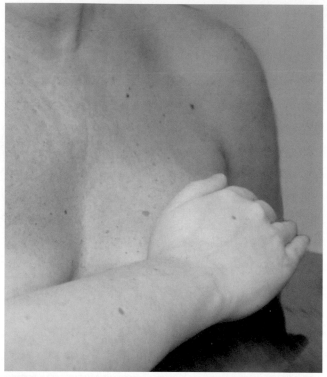

Fig. 5.8 Hold the breast firmly in position before applying compression.

c. The breast is correctly positioned, ready for full compression immediately before making the exposure (Fig. 5.10).

Remember:

- Control the body and the breast until compression is complete.
- Expose immediately.
- Compression automatically releases as soon as exposure has terminated.

The CC should demonstrate:

- The nipple in profile and pointing toward the center of the long axis of the image.
- The majority of medial tissue.
- The majority of the lateral tissue with the exclusion of the axillary tail.
- Pectoral muscle demonstrated at the center of the film on approximately 30% of individuals.
- The distance from the nipple to chest wall should be comparable with the MLO projection. There should be no more than 1cm difference.

The breast in the CC position is shown in Fig. 5.11 and the resulting mammogram in Fig. 5.12.

THE MEDIOLATERAL OBLIQUE PROJECTION

The technique described is a structured approach to the MLO projection (Fig. 5.13) which breaks down each movement in order that the mammographer is able to maximize the chances of producing a high-quality mammogram.

The advantages of the technique described are:

- The demonstration of the inframammary angle, frequently an area of difficulty for the mammographer, is given high priority.

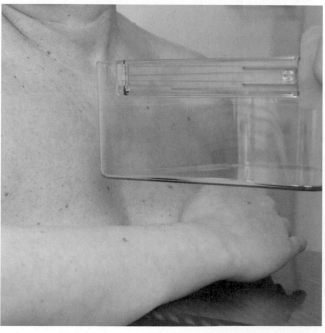

Fig. 5.9 Maintain the forward pull as compression is applied.

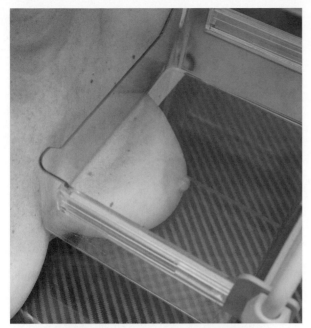

Fig. 5.11 Breast in craniocaudal position.

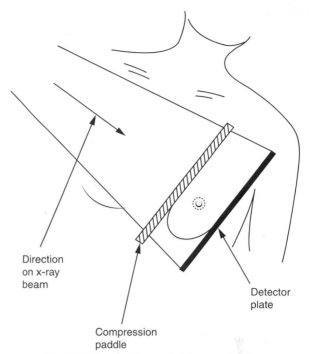

Direction
on x-ray
beam

Detector
plate

Compression
paddle

Fig. 5.13 The mediolateral oblique projection.

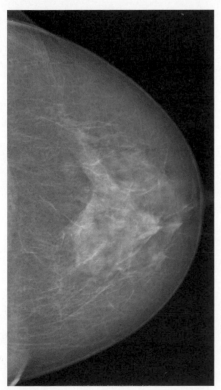

Fig. 5.12 The craniocaudal mammogram.

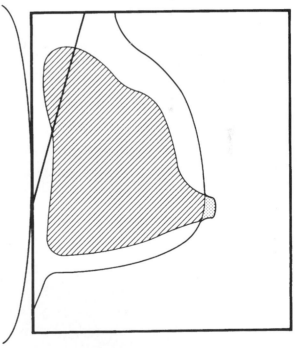

Fig. 5.14 The area demonstrated.

- Skin folds in the axillary region are eliminated.
- The complex movement required to place the axilla accurately can be fully explained to the trainee mammographer.

Area Demonstrated

Carefully performed, the MLO is the only projection in which all the breast tissue can be demonstrated on one image, from the inferior mammary angle to the superior border of the breast and from the nipple to the pectoral muscle deep to the posterior border of the breast (Fig. 5.14).

Equipment Position

The machine should be rotated according to the stature of the woman, usually between 40 and 55 degrees. The top of the detector plate should be level with the notch beneath the clavicle and humeral head when the woman's arm is by her side.

Anatomic Position: Left Breast

The woman faces the machine with her feet pointing toward the machine. The lateral edge of the thorax should be in line with the edge of the detector plate (Fig. 5.15). The mammographer should stand slightly behind and to the right of the woman.

Breast Positioning

a. Ask the woman to place her left hand on her head and lift her chin up lengthening along the lateral edge of the breast (Fig. 5.16).

b. Lifting the breast with the right hand, guide the woman into the machine (Fig. 5.17).

c. Keeping the nipple in profile, encourage her to lean forward into the machine, and then slightly laterally. Using the light beam diaphragm, check that the nipple is still in profile (Fig. 5.18).

d. To ensure the whole breast is imaged, the inframammary angle must be seen on the detector plate (Fig. 5.19).

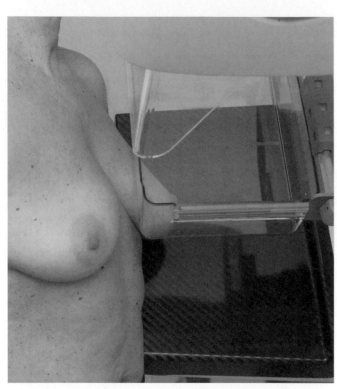

Fig. 5.15 Preparing for the mediolateral oblique projection.

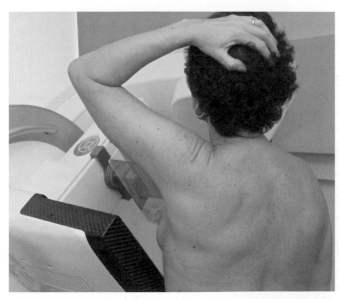

Fig. 5.16 Lengthening along the lateral edge of the breast.

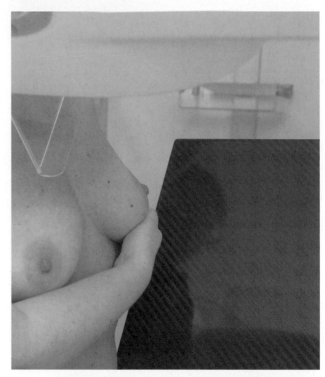

Fig. 5.17 Guide the woman into the machine.

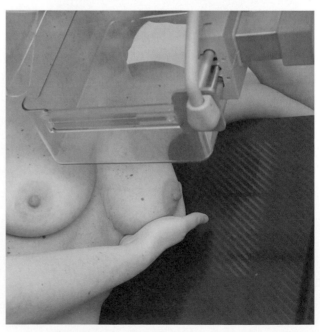

Fig. 5.18 Lift and guide the breast forward.

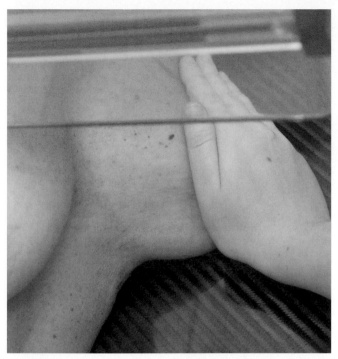

Fig. 5.19 Check the inframammary fold is fully visualized.

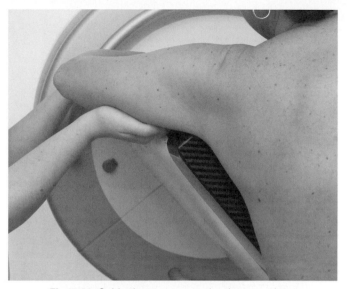

Fig. 5.20 Guide the arm across the detector plate.

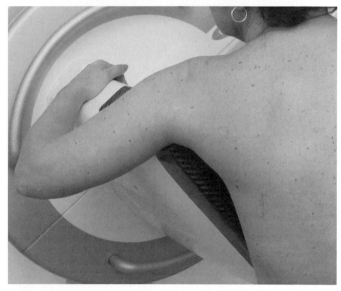

Fig. 5.21 Final resting place of the arm with the elbow relaxed.

If the criteria are not met, refer to Table 5.2.

e. When the nipple is in profile and the inframammary angle clearly demonstrated, go behind the detector plate, ensuring that the woman keeps her thorax in the same position.

f. Ask the woman to remove her hand from her head and guide her arm over the detector plate, being careful to not to take the weight of her arm. The corner of the detector plate will sit within her axilla (Fig. 5.20).

g. Continue to guide the arm across the corner, with the elbow slightly dropped behind the detector plate. At the same time, encourage her to relax her left shoulder.

h. Bring the woman's arm down, bending it so that she can rest her left hand on the machine in a comfortable position with the elbow hanging down behind the detector plate, with her hand resting on the detector plate (Fig. 5.21).

Remember:

• The breast and arm can be heavy and lifting should be avoided where possible, to achieve the best position, the mammographer should direct the woman through clear instruction to guide and control movement.

i. Ensuring that the woman does not move, return to the front of the detector plate. Run the fingers of the right hand along the back of the breast to check for creases in the axilla and at the lateral aspect of the breast (Fig. 5.22).

TABLE 5.2 Trouble Shooting		
Problem	**Cause**	**Corrective Action**
Nipple rotated toward detector plate	The woman's skin is caught on the detector plate at the lateral aspect	Lift the breast again and pull through at the lateral edge
Nipple rotated toward the tube	The hips and/or feet are rotated	Straighten the hips and feet so that they are pointing toward the machine
Inframammary angle not visualized	The hips and/or feet are rotated	Straighten the hips and feet so that they are pointing toward the machine
	The woman is standing too far behind the table	Encourage her to step toward you

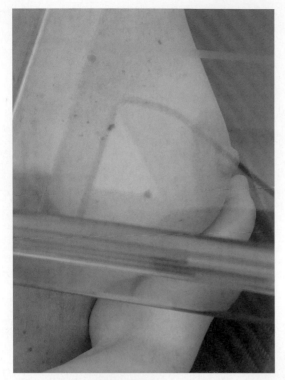

Fig. 5.22 Check for creases at the back of the breast and in the axilla.

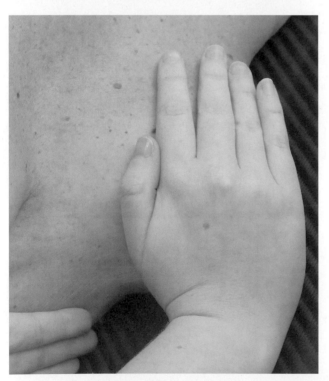

Fig. 5.23 Check for creases in the inframammary fold.

j. Check for potential creases at the inframammary fold (Fig. 5.23).

k. Once the inframammary fold is tidy, without creases, and lies fully on the detector plate, the breast is pulled away from the chest wall and held in position against the detector plate (Fig. 5.24).

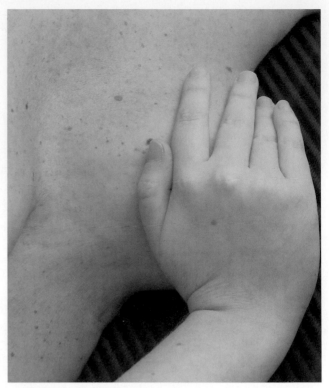

Fig. 5.24 Hold the breast firmly in position before applying compression.

l. Before applying compression, use the light beam diaphragm to check that the whole area to be imaged is included in the field of view as shown in Fig. 5.14.

   i. The pectoral muscle is across the detector plate by ensuring that the compression plate will be adjacent to the thorax from immediately beneath the clavicle to the inframammary angle

   ii. The nipple is in profile

   iii. The inframammary angle is clearly visible

There are no skin folds.

If criteria are not met, refer to Table 5.3.

Applying the Compression

a. Keep the shoulder relaxed on the detector plate. Maintaining the position of the breast away from the chest wall, using the palm of your right hand on the medial surface, pull gently forward toward the nipple, ready to apply compression. As the compression paddle approaches the breast, it needs to be close to the sternum to ensure the medial and posterior aspects of the breast are included (Fig. 5.25).

b. Using the foot pedal, apply compression evenly and slowly, gradually moving the hand forward, towards the nipple, maintaining position until the compression plate has taken firm hold of the breast. The left hand controls the tummy and the inframammary angle (Fig. 5.26).

Remember:

- The left hand guides the body
- The right hand controls the breast
- Acquire image immediately
- Compression automatically releases as soon as exposure has terminated

TABLE 5.3 Troubleshooting

Problem	Cause	Corrective Action
Pectoral muscle not across the detector plate	The detector plate may be too high	Reduce height of machine Guide arm across the detector plate again and resettle shoulder
Nipple no longer in profile and/or inframammary angle no longer demonstrated	The pectoral muscle has been taken too far across the detector plate, with the result that the woman has rotated her thorax and/or hips The detector plate may be too high, and the breast is taut	Readjust shoulder position so that the thorax and hips can be turned back into position Lower the detector plate so that the breast is relaxed
Folds at the inframammary angle	Overlap of lower border of breast and abdominal wall Compression will exaggerate this and push the inframammary angle off the image	Insert forefinger between detector plate and the lateral edge of the breast. Hook out surplus tissue and pull down and tuck behind the detector plate (see Figs. 5.22–5.24)
Folds across the axilla (rings of Saturn)	The detector plate may be too high so that excessive lift of the breast creates a crease The woman has large breasts with a pad of fat/breast tissue in the axillary tail	Lower the detector plate with the woman still in position Attempt to smooth out the skin surface as compression is applied, placing a finger at the lateral aspect of the breast and sweeping the skin surface upward Two views may be necessary (see Chapter 6)

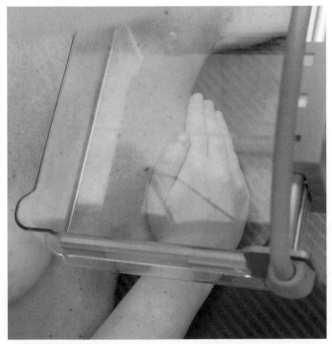

Fig. 5.25 Maintain the lift and forward pull of the breast while applying compression.

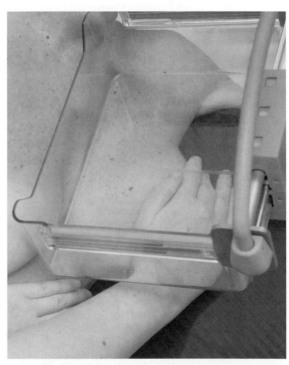

Fig. 5.26 Final position check before completing compression

The MLO mammogram should demonstrate:
- the inframammary fold
- the nipple in profile
- the nipple lifted to the level of the lower border of the pectoral muscle
- the pectoral muscle across the film at an appropriate angle for the individual woman (generally between 20 and 35 degrees from the vertical)

The final position is shown in Fig. 5.27 and the resultant mammogram in Fig. 5.28.

Difficulties With Even Application of Compression

It is not infrequent for novice mammographers to experience difficulties with applying compression. The compression paddle holds the axilla, but the breast itself droops. This is

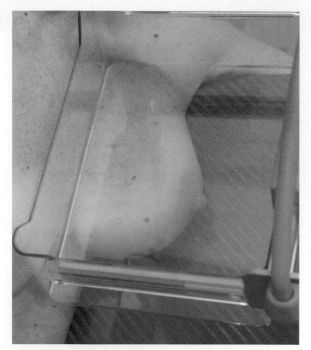

Fig. 5.27 Breast in the mediolateral oblique position.

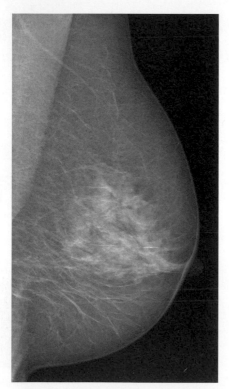

Fig. 5.28 The mediolateral oblique mammogram.

In some cases, supplementary views may be necessary to demonstrate all of the breast tissue (see Chapter 6).

The compression paddles on more modern equipment reduce uneven compression with designs such as curved paddles, shifting paddles, or flexible attachments which can be beneficial to the mammographer and the woman.

Adjusting to the Individual

To facilitate accurate positioning in the MLO position, consideration of the woman's anatomy must be taken. The reasons behind this are fully explained in Chapters 3 and 7.

However, as a general rule, if a woman has narrow shoulders with small breasts, a slightly steeper angle of 50 to 55 degrees from the horizontal should be selected, if accurate positioning proves difficult.

In the case of a woman with broad shoulders, a flatter angle of 40 degrees from the horizontal may prove more successful.

FURTHER READING

Andolina, V. (2011). *Mammographic imaging: a practical guide* (3rd ed.). Philadelphia: Wolters Kluwer/Lippincott Williams & Wilkins Health.

Dumky, H., Leifland, K., Fridell, K. (2018). The art of mammography with respect to positioning and compression—A Swedish perspective. *Journal of Radiology Nursing,* 37(1), 41–48.

Harvey, J., March, D.E. (2013). *Making the diagnosis: a practical guide to breast imaging.* Philadelphia: Saunders Elsevier.

Hogg, P., Kelly, J., Mercer, C. (2015). *Digital Mammography* (eds.). Springer International Publishing.

Huppe, A.I., Overman, K.L., Gatewood, J.B., Hill, J.D., Miller, L.C., Inciardi, M.F. (2017). Mammography positioning standards in the digital era: Is the status quo acceptable? *American Journal of Roentgenology,* 209(6), 1419–1425.

Kopans, D.B. (2006). Breast Imaging (3rd ed). Baltimore, Maryland: Lippincott Williams & Wilkins.

Mackenzie, A., Warren, L.M., Wallis, M.G., et al. (2016). The relationship between cancer detection in mammography and image quality measurements. *Physica Medica,* 32(4), 568–574.

Nightingale, J.M., Murphy, F.J., Robinson, L., Newton-Hughes, A., Hogg, P. (2015). Breast compression – An exploration of problem solving and decision-making in mammography. *Radiography,* 21(4), 364–369.

Popli, M.B., Teotia, R., Narang, M., Krishna, H. (2014). Breast positioning during mammography: mistakes to be avoided. *Breast Cancer: Basic and Clinical Research,* 8(30), 119–124.

Public Health England. (2018). Breast screening mammography: ergonomics good practice. October. Available at: https://www.gov.uk/government/publications/breast-screening-ergonomics-in-screening-mammography/breast-screening-mammography-ergonomics-good-practice (Accessed 20/04/20).

Public Health England. (2017). NHS Breast Screening Programme Guidance for breast screening mammographers. 3rd Ed. Available at: https://assets.publishing.service.gov.uk/government/uploads/system/uploads/attachment_data/file/819410/NHS_Breast_Screening_Programme_Guidance_for_mammographers_final.pdf (Accessed 20/04/20).

a result of "bulk" at the axilla and frequently occurs with heavily built women.

To reduce this bulk, the axillary region should be repositioned so that the elbow hangs down behind the detector plate and the pectoral muscle is brought parallel to the detector plate. If the problem continues, the detector plate should be slightly lowered and the procedure repeated.

Reynolds, A. (2014). Quality assurance and ergonomics in the mammography department. Radiologic Technology, 86(1), 61M–79M.

Shetty, M.K. ed. (2014). *Breast cancer screening and diagnosis: a synopsis.* New York: Springer.

Sweeney, R.J.I., Lewis, S.J., Hogg, P., McEntee, M.F. (2018). A review of mammographic positioning image quality criteria for the craniocaudal projection. *British Journal of Radiology,* 91(1082), 41–48.

Tabar, L., Dean, P., Boulter, P. (2012). *Teaching atlas of mammography.* (4th ed). Stuttgart, Germany: Thieme Publishing Group.

Théberge, I., Guertin, M.-H., Vandal, N., et al. (2018). Clinical image quality and sensitivity in an organized mammography screening program. *Canadian Association of Radiologists Journal,* 69(1), 16–23.

6

Mammography: Complementary Projections

CHAPTER CONTENTS

OBJECTIVES

This chapter outlines:
- How to perform additional mammographic projections which may be required for assessment of a possible abnormality in the breast

- Evaluate the accuracy of positioning
- Localize lesions accurately for special procedures
- Image specimens of core-cut, Mammotome, and excision biopsies

COMMUNICATION

A fully cooperative woman makes the task of achieving high-quality mammography much easier. For localized views, it is helpful to explain:

- what is being attempted
- why it is being attempted
- that the procedure is not easy, and that the woman's assistance and cooperation is essential if satisfactory images are to be obtained (i.e., it is a team effort).

Most women respond well to being shown the images being involved in the task, whatever the outcome. The mammographer should always take care, however, that she does not give an indication of the probable interpretation of the investigation, whether benign or malignant. The mammographer should not interpret the films for the woman nor offer false reassurance.

MEDIALLY ROTATED CRANIOCAUDAL PROJECTION

Indications

This projection is indicated for:

- lesions demonstrated in the mediolateral oblique (MLO) but not on the craniocaudal (CC) projection,
- lesions located in the extreme lateral portion of the breast,
- large breasted women who require more than one film in the CC position.

Area Demonstrated

This projection shows the lateral and mid-line portions of the breast (Figs. 6.1 and 6.2).

Equipment Position

The detector plate is horizontal and raised to just above the level of the inframammary angle.

Anatomic Position: Left Breast

The woman faces the machine, about 5 to 6 cm back, with the feet turned 5 to 10 degrees to the right. The breast should be aligned slightly to the right of center of the table. Her head should be turned to the right (Fig. 6.3).

Breast Positioning

1. Lift the left breast with both hands, one on the medial breast and one on the lateral breast. Keeping her shoulder

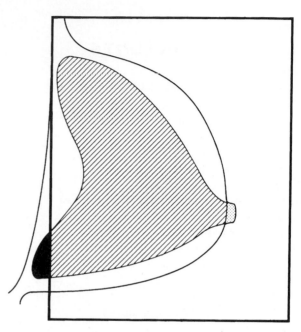

Fig. 6.2 The area demonstrated.

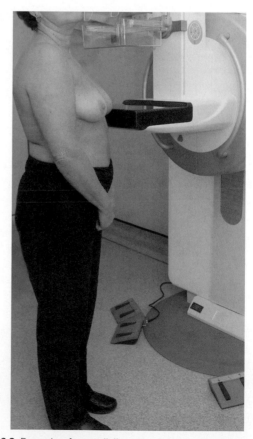

Fig. 6.3 Preparing for medially rotated craniocaudal projection.

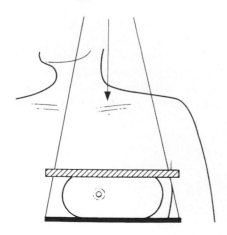

Fig. 6.1 The medially rotated craniocaudal projection.

relaxed. Pull the tissue firmly from the back of the breast (Fig. 6.4).

2. Encourage the woman to lean into the machine, bringing the lateral portion of the breast on to the image. The medial portion of the breast will not be on the image. Maintaining the relaxed shoulder, ensure the nipple is in profile, pointing slightly medial to the long axis of the detector plate and that there are no skin folds on the superior and inferior skin surfaces (Fig. 6.5).

3. Secure the breast with the palm, maintaining the forward pull on the lateral aspect of the breast; use the foot pedal to apply compression using the compression paddle to enhance this effect. Expose immediately (Fig. 6.6).

The final medially rotated CC position and resultant mammogram are illustrated in Figs. 6.7 and 6.8:
- the nipple points slightly medially,
- the muscle may be demonstrated, in the lateral portion of the breast.

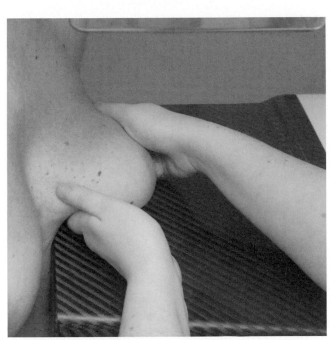

Fig. 6.4 Pull the tissue firmly from the back of the breast.

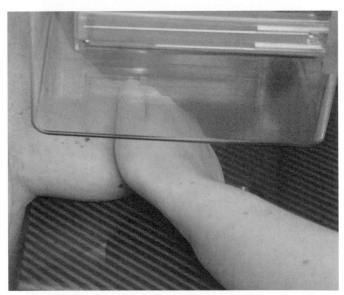

Fig. 6.6 Maintain the forward pull as compression is applied.

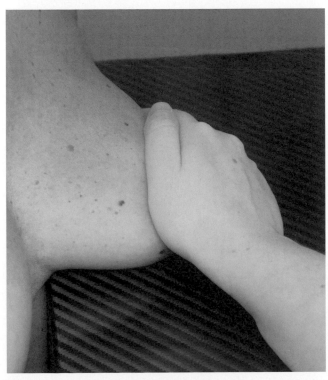

Fig. 6.5 Hold the breast firmly in position before applying compression.

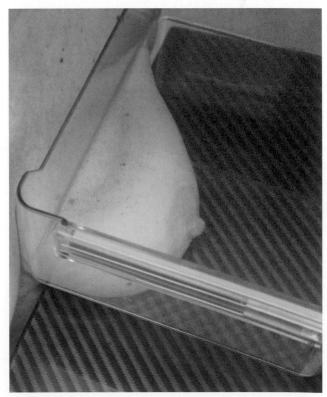

Fig. 6.7 Breast in the medially rotated craniocaudal position.

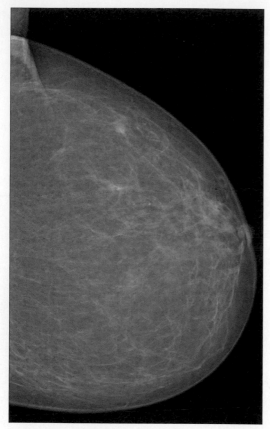

Fig. 6.8 The medially rotated craniocaudal mammogram.

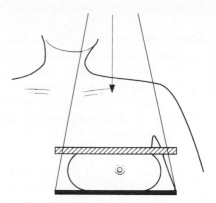

Fig. 6.9 The laterally rotated craniocaudal projection.

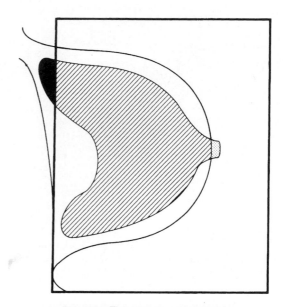

Fig. 6.10 The area demonstrated.

Difficulties Encountered

The head of the humerus may prevent clear imaging of the lateral aspect on some women. A suitable alternative would be the extended CC.

LATERALLY ROTATED CRANIOCAUDAL PROJECTION

Indications

Occasionally, a lesion may be demonstrated on the MLO which is not evident on the standard CC view. If the whole lateral aspect has been demonstrated on this view it is a possibility that the lesion lies medially.

Area Demonstrated

The extreme medial portion of breast and the skin over the sternum are shown (Figs. 6.9 and 6.10).

Equipment Position

The detector plate is horizontal and raised to just above the level of the inframammary angle.

Anatomic Position: Left Breast

The woman faces the machine, with her feet straight on, and her body as close as possible to the table. The breast should be aligned slightly right of center of the detector plate (Fig. 6.11).

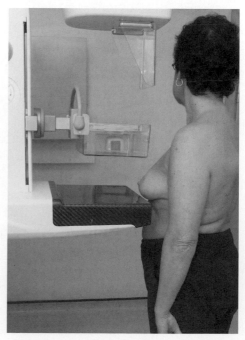

Fig. 6.11 Preparing to perform a laterally rotated craniocaudal projection.

Breast Positioning

1. Lift the left breast with both hands, one on the medial breast and one on the lateral breast. Keeping her shoulder relaxed, pull the breast tissue away from the chest wall (Fig. 6.12).
2. Lift the left breast, bringing the medial portion of the breast onto the detector plate (Fig. 6.13).
3. Lift the medial portion of the right breast on to the detector plate to prevent drag on the left breast and to aid demonstration of the cleavage (Fig. 6.14).

4. Encourage the woman to lean forward, and turn her head toward her left shoulder, so that it rests against the side of the face guard. Ensure that the medial portions of both breasts are pulled forward and fold free and that the sternum is against the detector plate. Put your left hand on the mid-dorsal area to maintain forward pressure. Keep the medial part of the breast pulled forward ready to apply compression (Fig. 6.15).

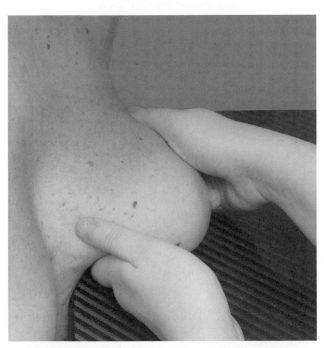

Fig 6.12 Pull the tissue firmly from the back of the breast.

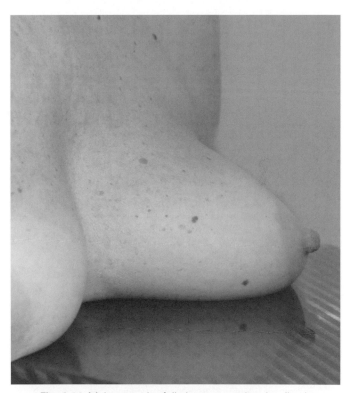

Fig. 6.14 Make sure the full cleavage can be visualized.

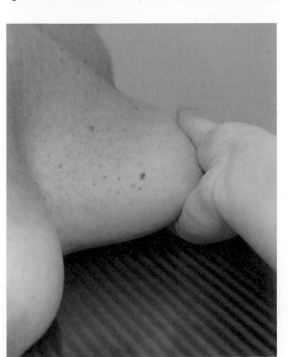

Fig. 6.13 Pull the medial edge of the breast onto the detector plate.

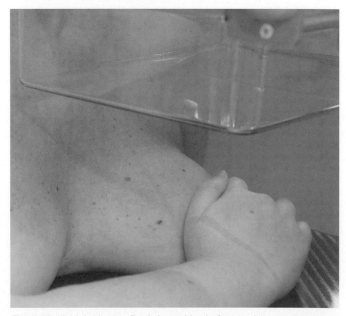

Fig. 6.15 Hold the breast firmly in position before applying compression.

5. Keeping medial portion of the left breast pulled forward with the right hand, use the foot pedal until fully compressed (Fig. 6.16). Expose immediately.

The final laterally rotated CC position and resultant mammogram are illustrated in Figs. 6.17 and 6.18:
- the nipple points slightly laterally,
- the cleavage may be demonstrated.

Difficulties Encountered

Imaging the medial portion of the breast can be difficult for the woman, as the tube housing may be in the way of their head. Encouragement may be required to optimize imaging.

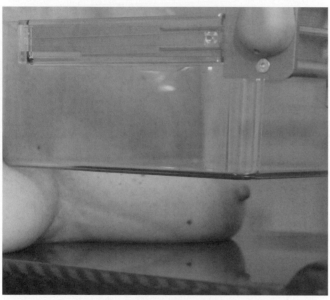

Fig. 6. 16 Full compression.

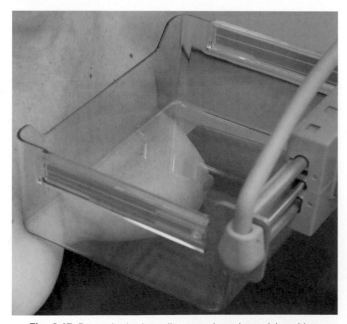

Fig. 6.17 Breast in the laterally rotated craniocaudal position.

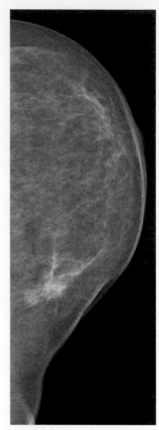

Fig. 6.18 The laterally rotated craniocaudal mammogram.

EXTENDED CRANIOCAUDAL PROJECTION

Indications

This projection is used to show a lesion seen high in the axillary tail on the MLO but not demonstrated on a CC.

Area Demonstrated

The axillary tail and upper midline portion of breast tissue are demonstrated (Figs. 6.19 and 6.20).

Equipment Position

The machine should be rotated 5 to 10 degrees from the horizontal at the lateral aspect (Fig. 6.21). It should be slightly below the level of the inframammary angle.

Anatomic Position: Left Breast

The woman should stand close to the machine with her breast aligned slightly right of center of the detector and their feet and hips pointing toward the machine.

Breast Positioning

a. Lift the left breast with both hands, one on the medial breast and one on the lateral breast. Keep the shoulder relaxed. Pull the breast tissue forwards and away from the chest wall; place on the detector plate (Fig. 6.22).

b. With the woman slightly turned, encourage her to lean 10 to 15 degrees to the lateral, extending her arm away from

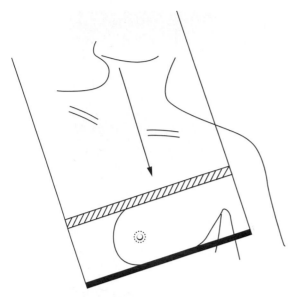

Fig. 6.19 The extended craniocaudal projection.

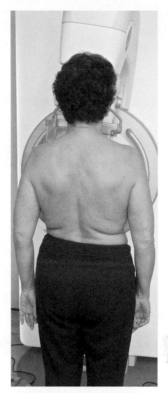

Fig. 6.21 Preparing to perform an extended craniocaudal projection.

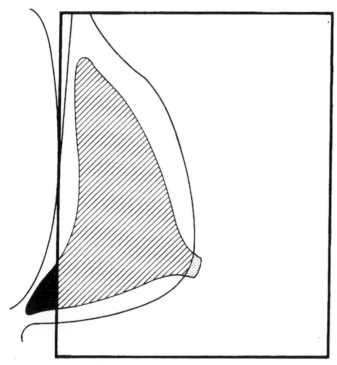

Fig. 6.20 The area demonstrated.

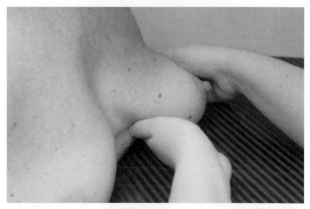

Fig. 6.22 Pull the tissue firmly from the back of the breast.

the side of her body, loosely holding the handle if she feels unsteady (Fig. 6.23).

c. While maintaining a slight turn and relaxed shoulder, keep the lateral aspect of the breast pulled forward and fold free (Fig. 6.24).

d. Put your right hand on the axillary tail area to maintain forward pressure as compression is applied. Once fully compressed expose immediately.

The final extended CC position and resultant mammogram are illustrated in Figs. 6.25 and 6.26.

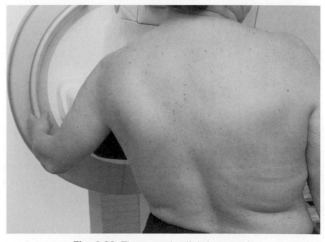

Fig. 6.23 The torso is slightly turned.

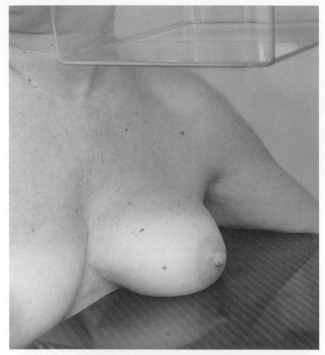

Fig. 6.24 Lower the shoulder toward the corner of the detector plate.

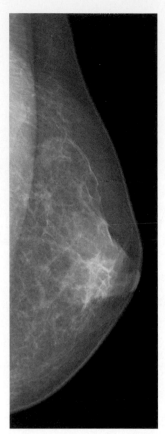

Fig. 6.26 The extended craniocaudal mammogram.

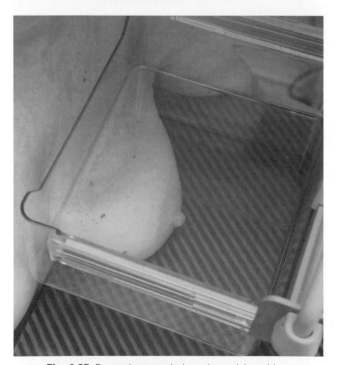

Fig. 6.25 Breast in extended craniocaudal position.

The extended CC projection should demonstrate:
- the nipple in profile
- the anterior edge of the pectoral muscle lateral to the midline of the breast.

Difficulties Encountered

This is an awkward position for the woman, and compression, exposure, and release should be accomplished with speed.

MEDIOLATERAL PROJECTION

Indications

This projection is indicated for the following:
- depth localization of lesions
- post stereotactic or ultrasound marker localization
- alternative view to clarify possible lesion demonstrated on MLO
- demonstration of the inframammary angle

Area Demonstrated

The majority of breast tissue with the exception of the axillary tail is viewed (Figs. 6.27 and 6.28).

Equipment Position

The detector plate is vertical.

Anatomic Position: Left Breast

The woman stands facing the machine with the lateral edge of her thorax in line with the detector plate. Her left arm should be relaxed by her side. The breast should be in line with the center of the light beam diaphragm (Fig. 6.29).

Breast Positioning

1. Ask the woman to place her left hand on her head and lift her chin up. Using your right hand, lift the breast up and away from the chest wall. Leading with the nipple, encourage her to lean forward into the machine (Fig. 6.30).

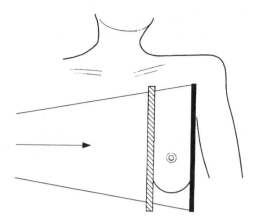

Fig. 6.27 The mediolateral projection.

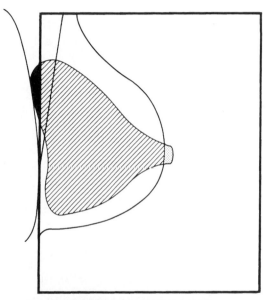

Fig. 6.28 The area demonstrated.

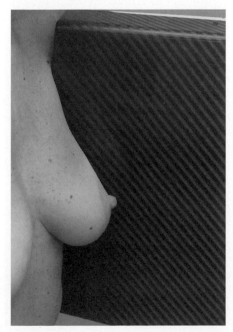

Fig. 6.29 Preparing to perform a mediolateral projection.

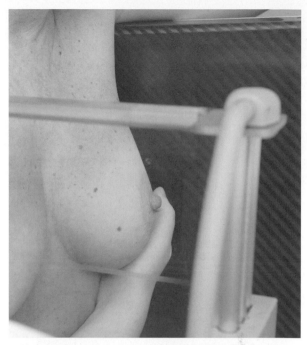

Fig. 6.30 Pull the tissue firmly from the back of the breast.

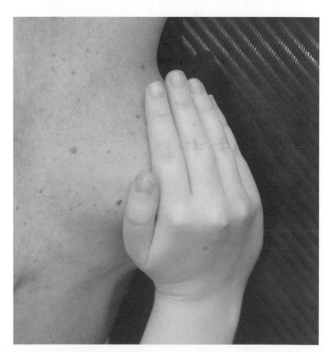

Fig. 6.31 Make sure the inframammary angle is fully pulled onto the detector plate.

2. Check that the nipple is in profile, and the inframammary angle is pulled onto the detector plate (Fig. 6.31).
3. Ask the woman to remove her hand from her head and guide her arm over the detector plate. Rest the woman's arm on top of the machine.
4. Using your right hand pull the upper portion of pectoral muscle forward onto the detector plate, ensuring that the corner is in the axilla (Fig. 6.32).
5. Using the right hand check that the corner of the detector plate is deep in the axilla (Fig. 6.33).

6. Holding the left breast in position, use the foot pedal to apply compression, and expose immediately.

The lateromedial position and resultant mammogram are illustrated in Figs. 6.34 and 6.35.

The mediolateral projection should demonstrate:

- the nipple in profile,
- the inframammary angle,
- the lower part of the pectoral muscle.

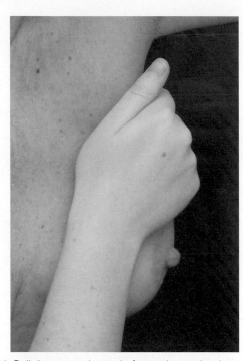

Fig. 6.32 Pull the pectoral muscle forward onto the detector plate.

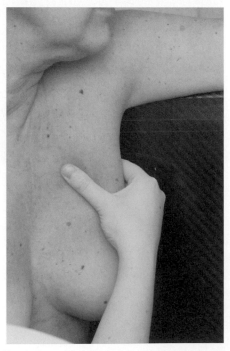

Fig. 6.33 Check the axillary tail is fully visualized with the corner of the detector plate tucked deep into the axilla.

Difficulties Encountered

Applying compression in lateromedial position is awkward for the mammographer because of the position of the tube housing. Removing the face shield or using a wheeled stool can help.

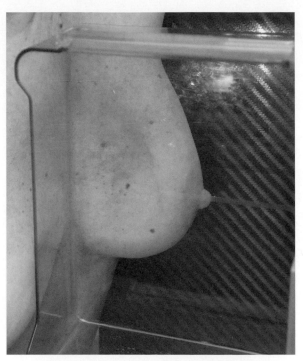

Fig. 6.34 Breast in the mediolateral position.

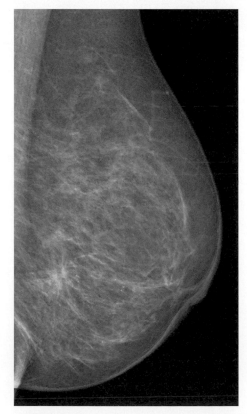

Fig. 6.35 The mediolateral mammogram.

LATEROMEDIAL PROJECTION

Indications

This projection is used in the following circumstances:
- to demonstrate the medial quadrants,
- to demonstrate the inframammary angle.

Area Demonstrated

The majority of breast tissue, excluding the axillary tail, is shown (Figs. 6.36 and 6.37).

Equipment Position

The detector plate is vertical.

Anatomic Position: Left Breast

The woman is erect and faces the machine, about 2 to 3 cm back, with the detector plate in line with her sternum (Fig. 6.38).

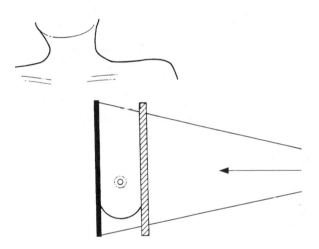

Fig. 6.36 The lateromedial projection.

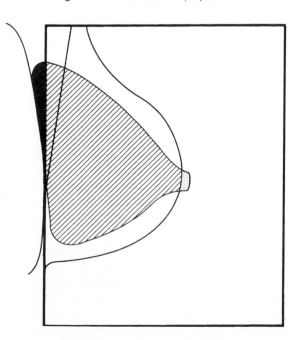

Fig. 6.37 The area demonstrated.

Breast Positioning

1. The woman should be asked to lift her left arm up and hold the support bar on the tube column, keeping her elbow slightly bent. Lift the left breast up and away from the chest wall with your left hand. Leading with the nipple, encourage her to lean toward the machine so that her sternum is against the detector plate (Fig. 6.39).
2. Encourage the woman to lean slightly to the medial and rest her forearm along the handlebar with the humerus parallel with the top of the detector plate. Check that the

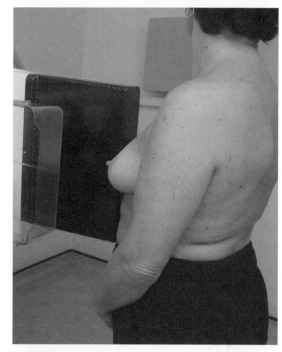

Fig. 6.38 Preparing to perform a lateromedial projection.

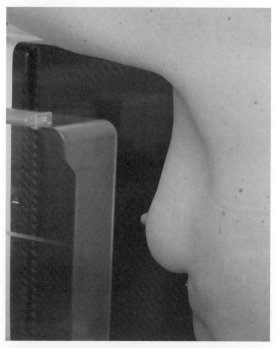

Fig. 6.39 The sternum is tight against the detector plate.

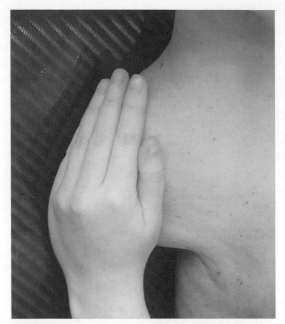

Fig. 6.40 Maintain the lift and forward pull of the breast before applying compression.

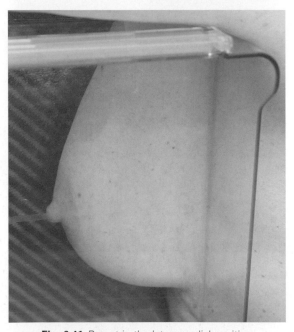

Fig. 6.41 Breast in the lateromedial position.

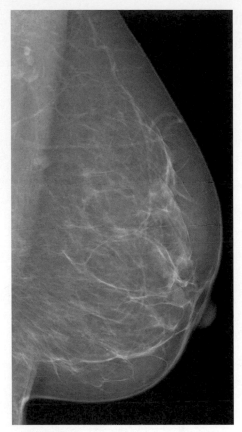

Fig. 6.42 The lateromedial mammogram.

inframammary angle and the anterior surface of the pectoral muscle are on the detector plate, and the nipple is in profile. Maintaining the lift and forward pull of the left breast with the left hand (Fig. 6.40), support the woman's back with the right hand, and using the foot pedal apply compression and expose immediately.

The lateromedial position and resultant mammogram are illustrated in Figs. 6.41 and 6.42.

Difficulties Encountered

Care must be taken that the compression paddle does not get caught on the edge of the posterior axillary fold.

AXILLARY TAIL VIEW

Indications

This projection is useful for woman with accessory breast tissue or the possibility of lymph gland involvement.

Area Demonstrated

The high axillary region is viewed (Figs. 6.43 and 6.44).

Anatomic Position: Left Breast

The woman should face the machine with her feet at an angle of approximately 15 degrees. She should stand close to the machine with her left hand on her head (Fig. 6.45).

Equipment Position

The gantry should be at 45 degrees from the horizontal and level with the notch beneath the end of the clavicle and the humeral head when the arm is raised.

Breast Positioning

1. Lean the woman forward toward the machine, placing the corner of the detector plate deep into the axilla (Fig. 6.46). Do not be concerned with the lack of inframammary angle.
2. From behind the detector plate, take hold of the woman's left arm and guide the arm and humeral head firmly across the top of the detector plate, ensuring that the corner is deep in the axilla (Fig. 6.47).

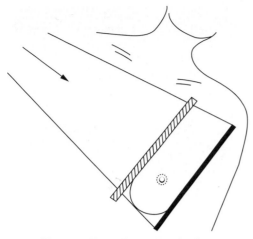

Fig. 6.43 The axillary tail projection.

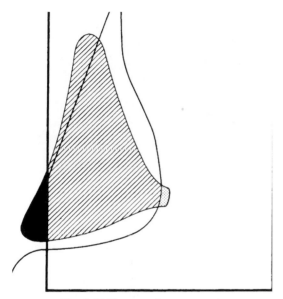

Fig. 6.44 The area demonstrated.

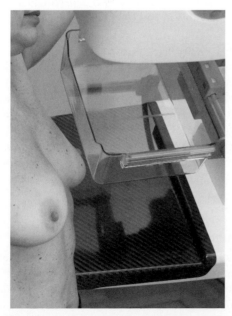

Fig. 6.45 Preparing to perform axillary tail view.

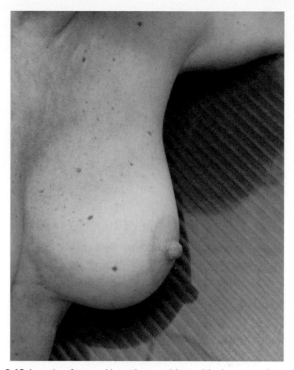

Fig. 6.46 Leaning forward into the machine with detector plate deep in the axilla.

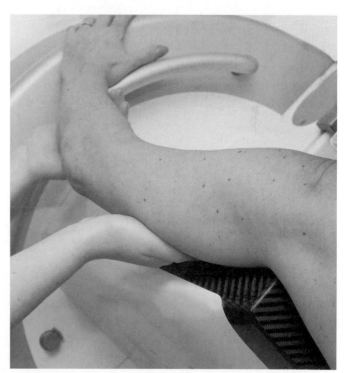

Fig. 6.47 Guide the arm across the top of the detector plate.

3. Returning to the front of the woman, hold the left breast forward with your right hand and ensure there are no folds (Fig. 6.48). Encourage her to rest onto the detector plate. With the foot pedal apply compression and expose immediately.

The axillary tail position and resultant mammogram are illustrated in Figs. 6.49 and 6.50.

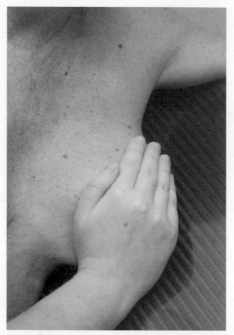

Fig. 6.48 Maintain the lift and forward pull of the breast before applying compression.

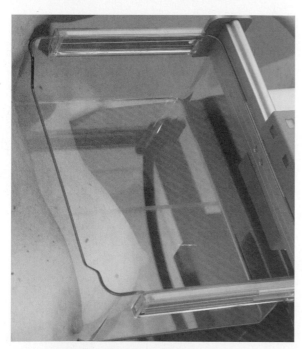

Fig. 6.49 Breast in axillary tail position.

Difficulties Encountered

Take care to avoid catching the humeral head or clavicle with the compression paddle.

SPECIALIZED TECHNIQUES

These techniques are used when the basic projections have indicated a possible abnormality within the breast which requires further evaluation. Special projections are normally

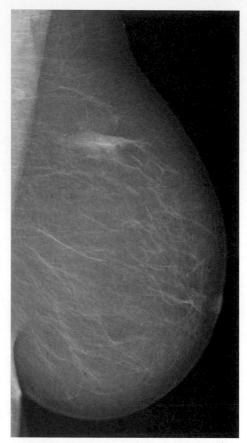

Fig. 6.50 The axillary tail mammogram.

requested by the responsible assessor (RA), but it is helpful for mammographers to have a full understanding of their uses. The RA may delegate the responsibility of deciding to undertake further views to the mammographer in his or her absence. An imaging department may have a set of work instructions in lieu of an RA. This will save the woman from having to make two visits to the department and the increased anxiety this provokes.

Equipment Required

Any equipment used for specialist techniques or additional view must meet the National Health Service Breast Screening Programme standards for mammography equipment, including:
- a variety of compression paddles (e.g., coned compression, magnification, shifting paddle, stereotactic paddle) (Fig. 6.51),
- a variety of pre- and postprocessing algorithms (three-dimensional [3D] mammography, two-dimensional [2D] mammography, implants, tomosynthesis, dual energy),
- supplementary equipment (stereotactic table, magnification table).

Positioning

Locating a small impalpable area in a large breast can be difficult. It must be recognized that time and care are required to minimize repeat images and associated stress levels for both woman and mammographer.

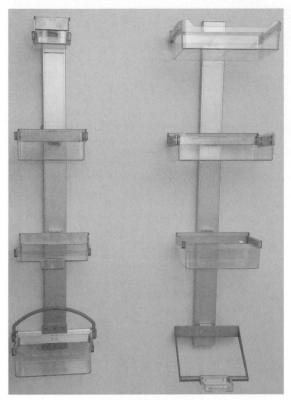

Fig. 6.51 A variety of compression paddles for different procedures.

ROLLED VIEWS/DISPLACEMENT VIEWS

Rolled views can be performed in any projection. They are most commonly used in the CC projection when superimposed tissue structures may be obscuring a lesion or may mimic a lesion. They can be a valuable alternative to paddle compression views which are explained in the section that follows. This technique can:

- project the superficial tissues away,
- expose the obscured areas,
- determine the reality of a lesion,
- demonstrate whether the lesion was superficial or deep.

A more acceptable technique might be to angle the tube 10 to 15 degrees which would reduce discomfort. When performing either rolled or displacement views the direction of roll, or tube swing, respectively, should be noted on the image.

LOCALIZED COMPRESSION OR "PADDLE" VIEWS

Indications

Paddle views are used:

- to demonstrate whether a lesion is genuine or simply superimposition of normal tissue and/or
- to demonstrate whether a lesion has clearly defined or ill-defined borders.

The RA will generally select the paddle views required but, in his/her absence, the paddle views should be performed in the positions which demonstrate the possible lesion.

Accurate Localization of the Area of Interest

In order to correctly locate a lesion, the mammographer should:

- examine the original medio-lateral/latero-medial and CC mammogram (Fig. 6.52)
- measure and note down:
  1. the depth of the lesion from the nipple back toward the chest wall,
  2. the distance of the lesion above or below nipple level (or medial/lateral to) (Fig. 6.52),
  3. the distance from the skin surface to the lesion.

Positioning

1. Position the woman mimicking, as closely as possible, the positioning on the original mammogram.
2. Referring to the noted coordinates, move the woman until the appropriate portion of breast tissue is centered under the small compression paddle in the respective views (Fig. 6.53). Remember to make allowances for the fact that your measurements are taken from a fully compressed breast.
3. Begin to apply the compression.
4. Once the breast is held in position, but not fully compressed, check the coordinates.
5. If you are satisfied that the area of interest is beneath the paddle:
   i. make a mark on the skin at the edge of the paddle,
   ii. apply compression fully and expose immediately.
6. If not, adjust the woman's position until you are satisfied.

Compression Force

With paddle views, more compression force than normal should be applied to the localized area (Fig. 6.54). If the technique and the reason for the procedure have been explained to the woman sufficiently well, she will usually tolerate this extra force.

Difficulties Encountered

If the area of interest is not central to the small paddle it may be pushed out of the image field. A second attempt will be necessary using the skin marks to guide the required adjustments.

MAGNIFICATION VIEWS

Indications

Digital imaging now allows electronic magnification of all or part of the breast and dedicated magnification views are less common in the digital age. They can be useful in the assessment of microcalcification, because of the higher resolution achieved. This allows more accurate assessment of the size, number and characteristic of the calcification.

Magnification views should be taken in the CC and lateral projections using dedicated accessories to standard equipment (Fig. 6.55). The latter will demonstrate the "teacup" effect typical of benign-type calcifications described in Chapter 11.

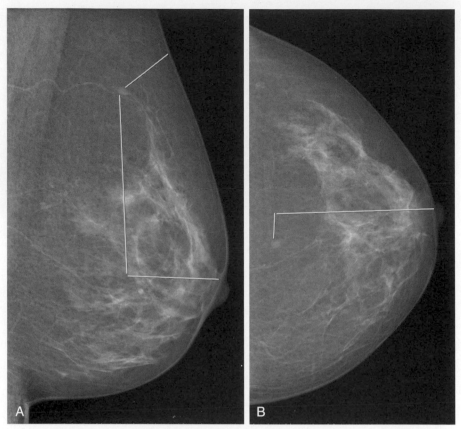

Fig. 6.52 Localizing a possibly abnormality, taking measurements for (A) the lateral position and (B) the craniocaudal position.

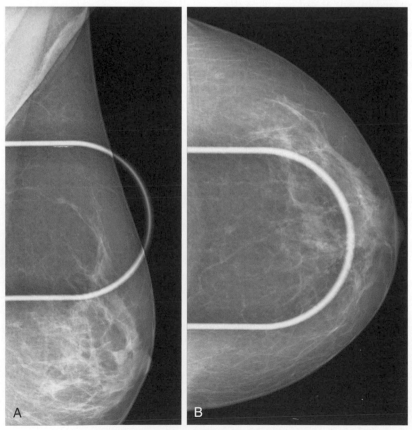

Fig. 6.53 "Paddle" in (A) lateral and (B) craniocaudal projections, confirming the presence of a mass.

LOCALIZED/PADDLE MAGNIFICATION VIEWS

Small paddle magnification is generally most helpful in that compression can be applied more vigorously to the area of interest, improving contrast and definition. The measuring and positioning technique used for standard paddle views should again be used to locate the area of interest with accuracy. However, in cases where the calcification is extensive, a larger compression paddle can be used to visualize the whole area on one image.

Exposure Time

Because of the use of fine focus, the exposure time will be considerably extended. It is advisable to ask the woman to stop breathing. (Note: do not ask the woman to breathe in and hold their breath. The expansion of the thorax will move the breast and your careful measuring will have been wasted!)

The final position is shown in Fig. 6.56 and the resultant mammogram in Fig. 6.57.

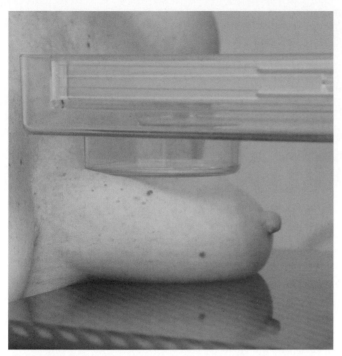

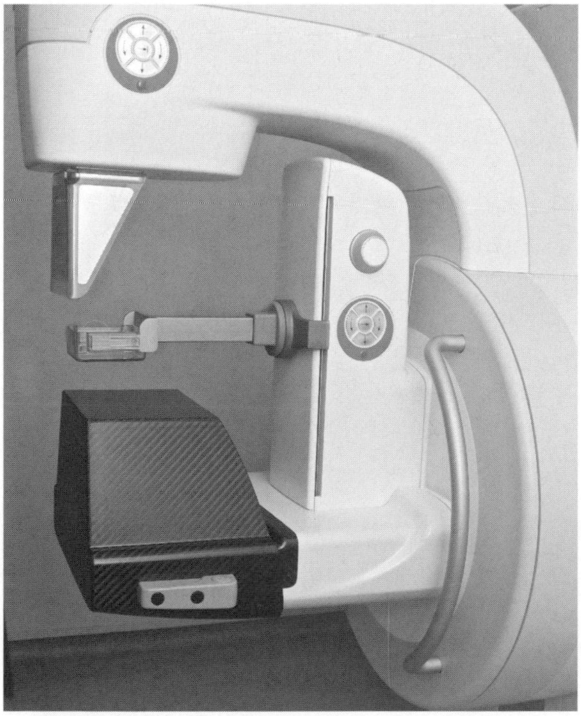

Fig. 6.54 The breast accurately positioned just before applying full compression.

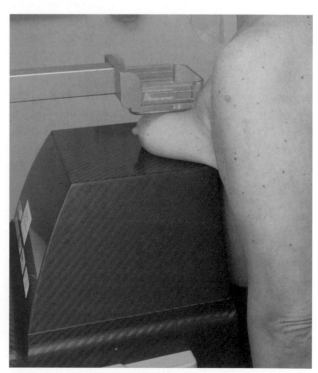

Fig. 6.55 Equipment for magnification projections.

Fig. 6.56 Final position just before applying full compression.

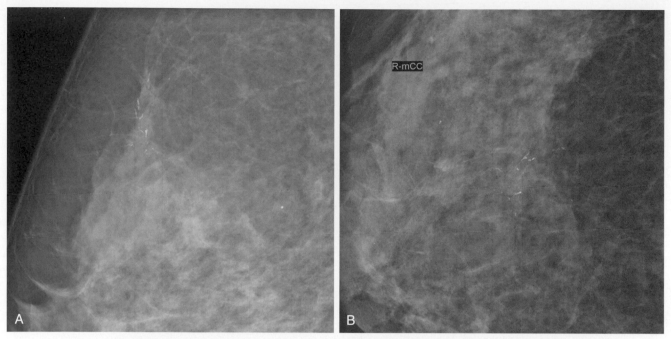

Fig. 6.57 Magnification views in (A) the lateral projection and (B) the craniocaudal projection.

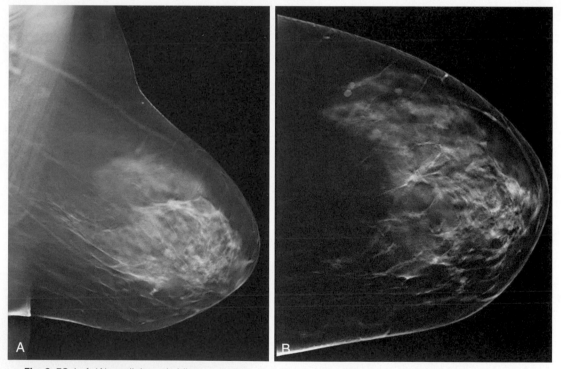

Fig. 6.58 Left (A) mediolateral oblique projection and (B) craniocaudal projection with digital breast tomosynthesis showing a "slice" through the breast.

DIGITAL BREAST TOMOSYNTHESIS

Digital breast tomosynthesis (DBT) uses the same technology as standard mammography. However, whereas standard mammograms are 2D and provide a flat image, tomosynthesis creates a 3D image. The techniques for positioning of the woman is the same as that for standard CC and MLO mammography but the patient must be advised that the x-ray tube will move above the breast and the exposure can take up to 10 seconds longer than the standard mammogram. The result is "slices" (Fig. 6.58) through the breast which can be viewed as individual images or used to reconstruct a 3D image. Some machines will create synthetic 2D standard mammograms.

CONTRAST ENHANCED DUAL-ENERGY MAMMOGRAPHY

For contrast enhanced dual-energy mammography (CEDM), positioning of the breast is as for standard CC and MLO mammography images (Fig. 6.59). The breast is subjected to low and high energy exposures pre- and postcontrast injection and a subtraction image is created. As breast cancers are vascular in nature the contrast is absorbed by the cancer and will be seen clearly on the subtraction image (Fig. 6.60).

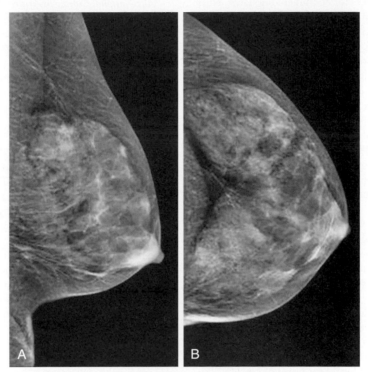

Fig. 6.59 Left breast two-dimensional (A) mediolateral oblique projection and (B) craniocaudal projection.

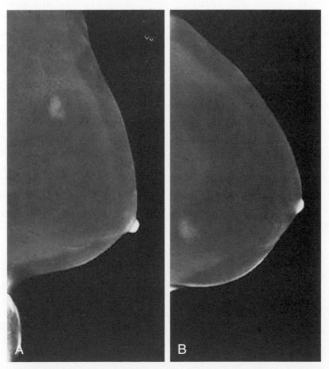

Fig. 6.60 Left breast contrast enhanced dual-energy mammography subtraction images (A) mediolateral oblique projection and (B) craniocaudal projection.

FURTHER READING

Andolina, V. (2011). *Mammographic imaging: a practical guide* (3rd ed.). Philadelphia: Wolters Kluwer/Lippincott Williams & Wilkins Health.

Barkhausen, J., Rody, A., Schafer, F.K.W. (2016). *Digital breast tomosynthesis: technique and cases.* New York: Thieme.

Baxter, G., Jones, V., Milnes, V., et al. (2014). NHS Cancer Screening Programmes Guidance notes for equipment evaluation and protocol for user evaluation of imaging equipment for mammographic screening and assessment. NHSBSP Equipment Report 1411. September. Public Health England. Available at: https://assets.publishing.service.gov.uk/government/uploads/system/uploads/attachment_data/file/442723/nhsbsp-equipment-report-1411.pdf (Accessed 20/04/20).

Borrelli, C., Cohen, S., Duncan, A., et al (2016). NHSBSP; Clinical guidance for breast cancer screening assessment, publication 49. Public Health England. Available at: https://associationofbreastsurgery.org.uk/media/1414/nhs-bsp-clinical-guidance-for-breast-cancer-screening-assessment.pdf (Accessed 20/04/20).

Covington, M.F., Pizzitola, V.J., Lorans, R., et al. (2018). The future of contrast-enhanced mammography. *AJR. American Journal of Roentgenology,* 210(2), 292.

Dromain, C., Balleyguier, C., Adler, G., Garbay, J.R., Delaloge, S. (2009). Contrast-enhanced digital mammography. *European Journal of Radiology,* 69(1), 34–42.

Feldman, E.D., Oppong, B.A., Willey, S.C. (2012). Breast cancer screening: clinical, radiologic, and biochemical. *Clinical Obstetrics and Gynaecology,* 55(3).

Giess, C.S., Frost, E.P., Birdwell, R.L. (2012). Difficulties and errors in diagnosis of breast neoplasms. *Seminars in Ultrasound, CT and MRI,* 33(4).

Gilbert, F.J., Tucker, L., Young, K.C. (2016). Digital breast tomosynthesis (DBT): a review of the evidence for use as a screening tool. *Clinical Radiology,* 71(2), 141-150.

Harvey, J., March., D.E. (2013). *Making the diagnosis: a practical guide to breast imaging.* Philiedelphia: Saunders Elsevier.

Hogg, P., Kelly, J., Mercer, C. eds (2015). *Digital mammography. a holistic approach.* Switzerland: Springer International Publishing.

Hooley, R.J., Durand, M.A., Philpotts, L.E. (2017). Advances in digital breast tomosynthesis. *American Journal of Roentgenology,* 208 (2).

Huppe, A.I., Overman, K.L., Gatewood, J.B., Hill, J.D., Miller, L.C., Inciardi, M.F. (2017). Mammography positioning standards in the digital era: Is the status quo acceptable? *American Journal of Roentgenology,* 209(6), 1419–1425.

Johnson, K., Sarma, D., Hwang, E.S. (2015). Lobular breast cancer series: imaging. *Breast Cancer Research,* 17(1), 94.

Kim, G., Phillips, J., Cole, E., et al. (2019). Comparison of contrast-enhanced mammography with conventional digital mammography in breast cancer screening: a pilot study. (Report). *Journal of the American College of Radiology,* 16(10), 1456.

Kopans, D.B. (2006). *Breast imaging* (3rd ed). Baltimore, Maryland: Lippincott Williams & Wilkins.

Mackenzie, A., Warren, L.M., Wallis, M.G., et al. (2016). The relationship between cancer detection in mammography and image quality measurements. *Physica Medica,* 32(4), 568–574.

Marinovich, M.L., Hunter, K.E., Macaskill, P., Houssami, N. (2018). Breast cancer screening using tomosynthesis or mammography: a meta-analysis of cancer detection and recall. *JNCI: Journal of the National Cancer Institute,* 110(9), 942–949.

Nightingale, J.M., Murphy, F.J., Robinson, L., Newton-Hughes, A., Hogg, P. (2015). Breast compression – An exploration of problem solving and decision-making in mammography. *Radiography,* 21(4), 364–369.

Nori, J, Kaur, M. (2018). *Contrast-enhanced digital mammography (CEDM).* Springer International.

Philpotts, L.E., Hooley, R.J. (2017). *Breast tomosynthesis.* Philadelphia: Elsevier.

Popli, M.B., Teotia, R., Narang, M., Krishna, H. (2014). Breast positioning during mammography: Mistakes to be avoided. *Breast Cancer: Basic and Clinical Research,* 8(30), 119–124.

Public Health England. (2017). NHS Breast Screening Programme Guidance for breast screening mammographers. 3rd Ed. Available at: https://assets.publishing.service.gov.uk/government/uploads/system/uploads/attachment_data/file/819410/NHS_Breast_Screening_Programme_Guidance_for_mammographers_final.pdf (Accessed 20/04/20).

Public Health England. (2018). Breast screening mammography: ergonomics good practice. October. Available at: https://www.gov.uk/government/publications/breast-screening-ergonomics-in-screening-mammography/breast-screening-mammography-ergonomics-good-practice (Accessed 20/04/20).

Reynolds, A. (2014). Quality assurance and ergonomics in the mammography department. *Radiologic Technology,* 86(1), 61M–79M.

Shetty, M.K. ed. (2014). *Breast cancer screening and diagnosis: a synopsis.* New York: Springer.

Sonnenschein, M., Waldherr, C. (2017). *Atlas of breast tomosynthesis.* Switzerland: Springer International Publishing.

Spuur, K., (2019). A review of mammographic lesion localisation and work up imaging in Australia in the digital era. *Radiography,* 25(4).

Tagliafico, A., Houssami, N., Calabrese, M. eds., (2016). *Digital breast tomosynthesis: a practical approach.* Switzerland: Springer.

Tennant, S.L., James, J.J., Cornford, E.J., et al. (2016). Contrast-enhanced spectral mammography improves diagnostic accuracy in the symptomatic setting. *Clinical Radiology,* 71(11), pp.1148-1155.

Travieso Aja, M.M., Rodríguez Rodríguez, M., Alayón Hernández, S., Vega Benítez, V., Luzardo, O.P. (2014). Dual-energy contrast-enhanced mammography. *Radiología* (English Edition), 56(5), 390–399.

Empty line

7

Mammography: Tailoring the Examination

CHAPTER CONTENTS

OBJECTIVES

This chapter outlines:
- The variations in women's anatomy
- How to adapt technique to accommodate variations
- Other modifications to consider

THE INDIVIDUAL

Mammography is a very intimate examination requiring the woman to be partially naked and the mammographer to handle the woman's breasts. Each woman/mammographer interaction will result in a unique examination/experience which is tailored to the individual. Body shape, height, habitus, anxiety and embarrassment may all be contributing factors to the quality of the resultant images. Some examinations are technically and physically more demanding for the woman and/or the mammographer and adaptations may need to be made to the standard techniques to obtain the best possible images for any given woman. Experience and the ability to adapt will help the mammographer accomplish high quality images in the majority of cases.

This chapter provides some guidance on how to approach physical characteristics which may compromise the mammographer's ability to demonstrate all of the breast tissue. Every woman has their own individual needs and it is down to the mammographer's' skill to accomplish an adequate examination, bearing in mind the need to demonstrate all areas of the breast.

Should an adequate examination not be achieved after every effort has been made, the mammographer should advise the reader of the difficulties and that the whole breast may not have been imaged. This is known as a partial mammography examination.

VARIATIONS IN BREAST DEVELOPMENT

The stereotypical breast (Fig. 7.1) is not the reality for most women who present in a wide variety of shapes and sizes (Fig. 7.2).

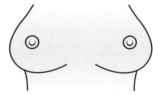

Fig. 7.1 Symmetrical breasts of even size and shape.

Variations	Description	Hints and tips
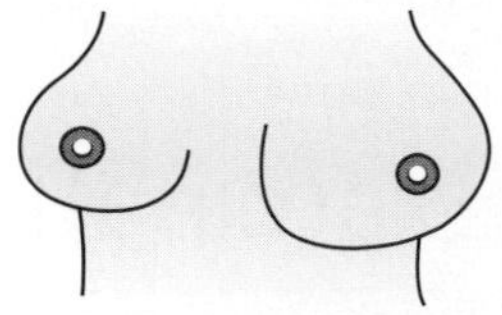 Asymmetrical breasts	Difference in size and shape of the breasts may need different techniques for each breast.	The resultant images may give the impression that breast tissue is missing. Make a note on the paperwork to avoid technical recalls.
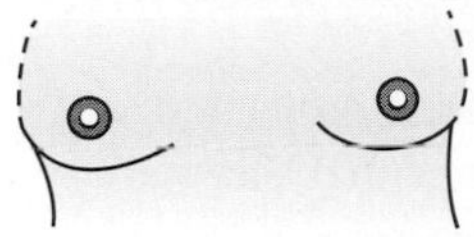 Low volume of breast tissue	Smaller breasts with a low volume of breast tissue	It may be difficult to control the breast tissue during compression. A smaller compression paddle may help. Care should be taken to ensure tissue covers the superpixel or in some cases a manual exposure may be required.
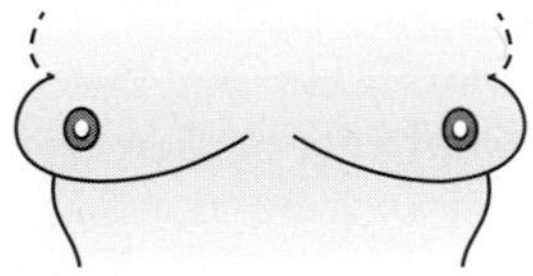 Athletic	Immobile, firm breast tissue closely attached to the chest wall.	It may be difficult to move the tissue away from the chest wall. A steeper angle may make it easier to visualize all of the tissue.
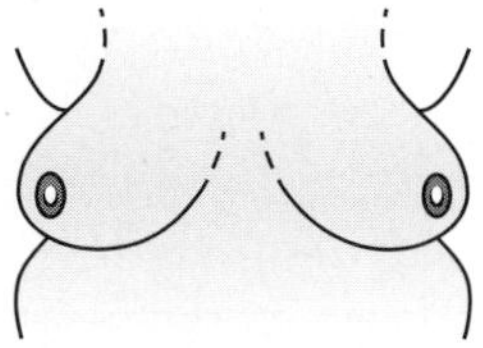 Pendulous/bell shaped	Heavy breast tissue with loose flesh at the top and increased volume of breast tissue hanging low on the chest wall. Will easily pull away from the chest wall	It may be difficult to control the breast tissue as the breasts may be heavy. Compression may be difficult to apply evenly. Care should be taken to reduce the risk of folds where the tissue is slack. Multiple images may be needed to include the whole breast. Women may have increased soreness under their breasts.
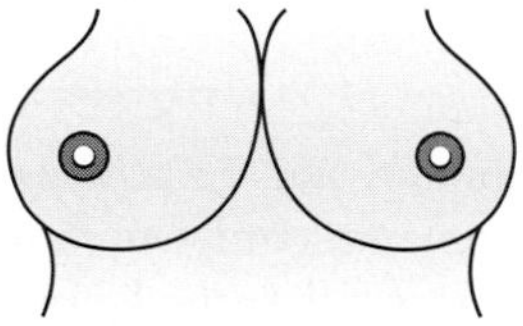 Frontal/close together	Firm rounded breasts with minimal room between the breasts, quite tight to the chest wall	It may be difficult to separate the breasts. It may be necessary to ask the women to hold her other breast out of the field of view. Beware of artefacts on the images, such as shadows from the other breast or fingers.
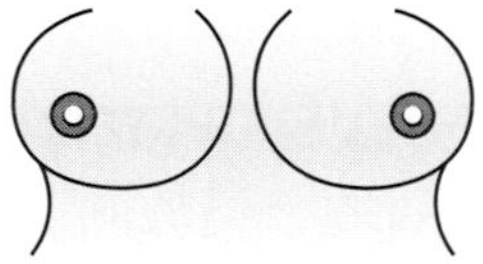 Ball shaped/immobile	Ball shaped breasts fairly immobile and tight to the chest wall.	Compression may be difficult to apply evenly. Breath holding may be helpful.
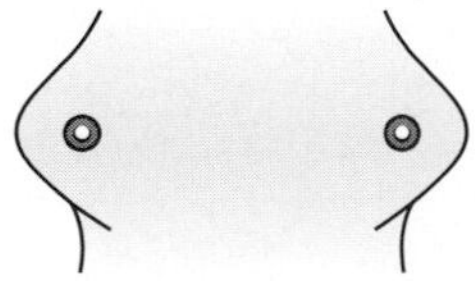 Cone shaped	Laterally placed breasts with a wide gap between with breast tissue bulging toward the sides of the chest wall	It may be difficult to get the nipple in profile; nipple views may be required. Care should be taken to ensure the lateral breast is pulled around into the field of view.

Fig. 7.2 Variation in breast shape; their technical challenges and considerations.

Variations	Description	Hints and tips
Involuted breasts—slack tissue with nipples downward direction	Loose breast tissue with the breast tissue pulling down and away from the chest wall, nipples pointing toward the floor. Fairly even volume of breast tissue.	It may be difficult to get the nipple in profile; nipple views may be required. Compression may be difficult to apply if there is very little breast tissue. Care should be taken to reduce the risk of folds where the tissue is slack.
Loose breast bottom heavy	Loose breast tissue but with more volume of breast tissue in the lower portion of the breast compared with the upper half.	Compression may be difficult to apply evenly if there is significantly more tissue in the lower breast. Care should be taken to reduce the risk of folds where the tissue is slack.
Externally rotated	The nipples pointing outwards away from the chest wall	It may be difficult to get the nipple in profile; nipple views may be required. Angling the torso slightly might be helpful.
Bottom heavy nipple superior	Rounded breasts that are heavier in the lower part with nipple quite high on the breast.	It may be difficult to get the nipple in profile; nipple views may be required. Compression may be difficult to apply evenly. Breath holding may be helpful.
Top heavy breasts with nipples lower half pointing inferiorly	Rounded breasts with a higher volume of breast tissue in the upper part of the breasts and the nipple on the lower part of the breast.	It may be difficult to get the nipple in profile; nipple views may be required. Compression may be difficult to apply evenly. Breath holding may be helpful.

Fig. 7.2, cont'd

Women will fall into one or more of the breast shapes shown in Fig. 7.2. The mammographer will need to adapt their technique to accommodate the variations to fully visualize the breast tissue. As mammography equipment is designed to perform high volume standard images, it will require an adaption of technique and supplementary views for some women. Supplementary views are a slight adaption to the standard views when it is not possible to demonstrate all of the breast tissue on the standard four views; these should not be confused with repeat views or complementary projections.

Each different shaped breast will be associated with its own set of challenges and the ability to adapt the technique is a sign of a skilled mammographer.

For some shaped breasts, for example, bottom heavy breasts with superior nipples, it may be difficult or not possible to get the nipple in profile and an anterior view in one or both projections may be required. For some shapes, it may be difficult to get full or even compression across the breast tissue, for example, ball shaped immobile breasts or where there is a larger volume of tissue in either the top or bottom half of the breast.

The heavy part of the breast must be placed centrally between the compression paddle and the detector plate to ensure that the compression maintains the breast in the correct position. In the mediolateral oblique (MLO) projection, in particular, if the center of the paddle makes contact above the center of the breast disc, the compression will push one portion of the breast off the detector. The inframammary fold is most commonly affected, as this is the point of least resistance.

Excessive compression on this type of breast, however well positioned, will ultimately push the breast out of the machine. The result is that insufficient length of pectoral muscle may be demonstrated.

For other shapes it may not be possible to visualize the inframammary fold or the lateral or medial border of the breast in one view.

Size Variation and Adapting Technique

The Smaller Breast

Small breasts or breasts with limited volume of tissue can be difficult to image satisfactorily but some simple small changes in technique can be very effective in helping to achieve diagnostic images. The secret is in the selection of the correct angle and height of the detector plate. Some manufacturers provide a slim compression paddle which can be useful when the breasts are particularly small.

Craniocaudal projection. Angling the detector by 5 to 10 degrees at the lateral aspect may help to visualize the axillary tail.

Mediolateral oblique projection. The secret to performing a good quality MLO on a smaller breast is the height of the machine. Any tension on the pectoral muscle (because of the detector plate being high or anxiety on the woman's part) will make positioning very difficult. On rare occasions, it may be necessary to use a manual exposure. Consideration must also be given to the appropriate angle for each individual.

Figs. 7.3 and 7.4 are mammograms of the same woman. Comparing the two, it is obvious that the image in Fig. 7.4 is significantly better; the improved image was achieved by adapting the positioning of the woman and correct selection of the machine height and angle.

The Larger Breast

No matter the size or shape of the breast, care is needed to ensure that all the breast is demonstrated on each projection. The technique for imaging any breast will vary according to breast size and stature of both the woman and the mammographer. In some cases, this may require more than one image with some degree of overlap on each image. This overlap should be kept to 5 to 6 cm to minimize repeated irradiation to one or other portion of the breast.

Care must be taken when underbreast soreness is present to avoid skin tears.

Craniocaudal projection

1. Stand the woman some 7 to 10 cm from the machine.
2. Ask the woman to stand up as straight and as tall as possible.

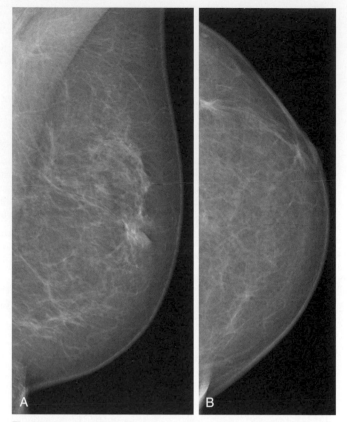

Fig. 7.3 Poorly positioned woman with breast missing (A) posteriorly and (B) laterally.

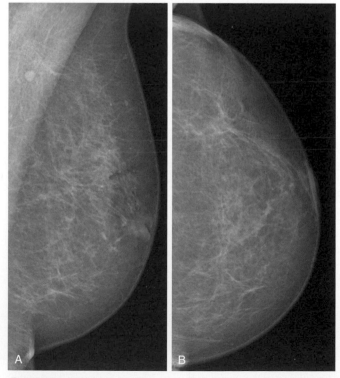

Fig. 7.4 By adapting the technique the whole breast is now imaged (A and B).

3. These two maneuvers help to lift the breast away from the abdomen and make good positioning easier.
4. Lift the breast in the normal way onto the detector plate.

If the breast is wide or the medial or lateral edge cannot be demonstrated on one image, imaging should consist of:

- A medially rotated craniocaudal (CC) projection (see Chapter 6) (Fig. 7.5)
- A laterally rotated CC projection (Fig. 7.6)

In each projection, attempt to have the nipple in profile.

If the breast is long, imaging should include:

- A posterior CC projection
- An anterior CC projection to include the nipple in profile (Fig. 7.7)

When the breasts are very large, imaging should include:

- A laterally rotated CC projection
- A medially rotated CC projection
- A nipple view

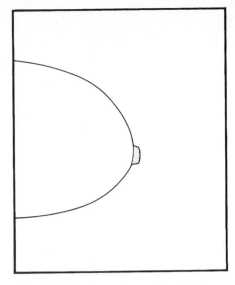

Fig. 7.7 Anterior craniocaudal projection.

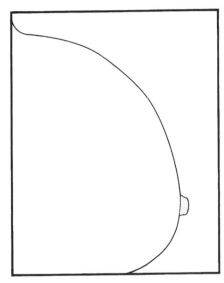

Fig. 7.5 Medially rotated craniocaudal projection.

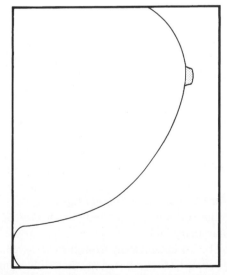

Fig. 7.6 Laterally rotated craniocaudal projection.

Mediolateral Oblique Projection. The technique is as follows:

1. Stand the woman 7 to 10 cm from the machine.
2. Ask her to stand as straight and tall as possible.
3. Adjust the height of the gantry in the usual manner (see Chapter 5).
4. Ask her to put her hand on her head.
5. Encouraging her to extend the lumbar region, and leading with the nipple, lean her into the machine.
6. Place her arm in the usual manner (see Chapter 5), taking particular care to eliminate excess skin and fat from the axillary region.
7. Lifting the breast up and away from the chest wall, examine the region of the inframammary fold.

If the breast is deep from clavicle to inframammary and the inframammary fold and lower border of the breast are excluded from the field, or the inframammary fold cannot be demonstrated on one image imaging should include:

- A superior MLO (Fig. 7.8)
- An inferior MLO (Fig. 7.9)

If the breast is long from the chest wall to the nipple and the inframammary fold and lower border are in the field, imaging should consist of:

- A posterior MLO (Fig. 7.10)
- An anterior MLO (Fig. 7.11)

When the breasts are very large imaging should consist of:

- A superior oblique
- An inferior oblique
- An anterior view to include the nipple in profile (see Fig. 7.11)

Superior Mediolateral Oblique Projection. Continuing from point 7 earlier, the technique is as follows:

8. Further extending her lumber region, withdraw the inframammary region and abdominal wall from the field.
9. Check for creases at the lateral border.
10. Lifting the breast up and away from the chest wall, spread the breast tissue across the film.

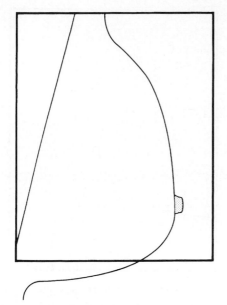

Fig. 7.8 Superior mediolateral oblique projection.

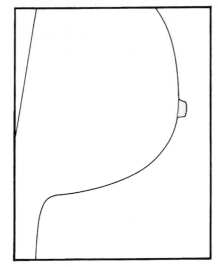

Fig. 7.9 Inferior mediolateral oblique projection.

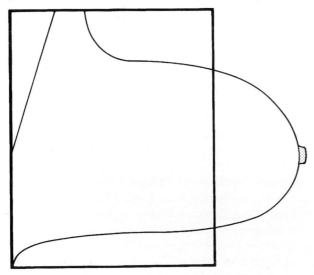

Fig. 7.10 Posterior mediolateral oblique projection.

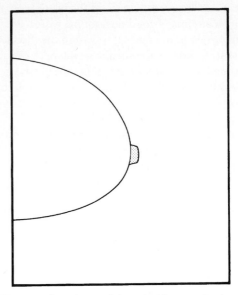

Fig. 7.11 Anterior mediolateral oblique projection.

11. Check that the nipple is in profile.
12. Apply compression in the usual way, taking care that the breast tissue is compressed effectively.

If difficulties are encountered, adjust the position of the axilla to reduce the bulk of tissue.

Inferior Mediolateral Oblique Projection. Do not adjust the detector plate height.

13. Stand the woman close to the detector.
14. Leave her arm by her side.
15. Lift the breast up and away from the chest wall.
16. Leading with the nipple, lean the woman forward into the machine, keeping firm hold of the breast until the edge of the detector plate is at the mid-axillary line. Check that:
    a. The inframammary fold is clearly demonstrated
    b. The nipple is in profile
    c. There are no skin folds at the lateral aspect
17. Lift the breast up and away from the chest wall.
18. Remove excess abdominal tissue from the inframammary region, employing the technique described in Chapter 5 to tidy the inframammary fold.
19. Apply compression to the breast, maintaining control of the breast throughout.

    In the inferior breast technique, the compression force is used to enhance the "lift" of the breast, thus helping to eliminate folds at the inframammary fold. The main body of the lower portion of the breast should lie a little above the center of the detector.

Posterior Mediolateral Oblique Projection

20. Using the technique described in Chapter 5, tidy the inframammary fold.
21. Lift the breast up and away from the chest wall.
22. Apply compression, ensuring that the compression applies to the breast and not only at the axilla.

Anterior Mediolateral Oblique Projection

23. Stand the woman 7 to 10 cm back from the machine.
24. Ask her to hold the handlebar so that she is steady.
25. Lift the distal part of the breast onto the film with the nipple in profile, allowing 1-to 2-cm overlap on the previous images.
26. Apply compression with care as the force will be applied to the most sensitive area of the breast.

Area Demonstrated. The superior MLO projection should demonstrate:

- The pectoral muscle to nipple level
- The pectoral muscle at correct angle
- The nipple in profile

The inframammary fold is not required on this view and this helps in excluding abdominal wall skin folds.

The inferior MLO projection should demonstrate:

- The inframammary fold
- The nipple in profile
- The lower border of the pectoral muscle

The posterior MLO projection should demonstrate:

- The full length of pectoral muscle
- The pectoral muscle at the correct angle
- The inframammary fold
- The breast lifted with the ducts spread out and not drooping

Anterior MLO projection should demonstrate:

- The nipple in profile
- The anterior portion of the breast that is not visualized on the posterior view with some evident overlap

These projections can be utilized to ensure all of the breast is imaged for almost all shapes and sizes. Where it has not been possible to demonstrate all of the breast tissue and a large enough percentage of breast tissue is missing, the examination can be categorized as a partial examination. The woman made aware that her whole breast has not been seen.

Variations in the Chest Wall Skeleton
Prominent Sternum

When imaging a woman with a prominent sternum (Fig. 7.12), the MLO projection is not as difficult as commonly believed.

Frequently, the breasts are more laterally pointing than usual and thus if the mammographer allows the woman to rotate her thorax medially a little, still leading with the nipple, an excellent result can be achieved.

In severe cases, two views may be necessary:

- A superior MLO, demonstrating the axilla, pectoral muscle, upper outer quadrant and the superior portion of the upper inner quadrant (Fig. 7.13).

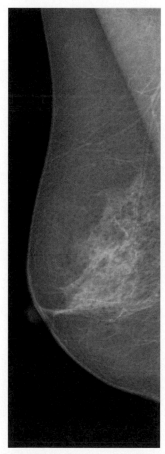

Fig. 7.13 Superior mediolateral oblique.

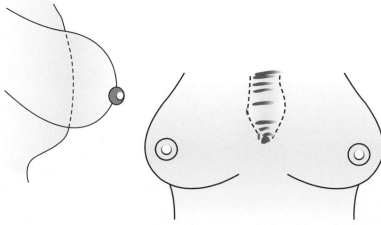

Fig. 7.12 The prominent sternum is convex in shape making it difficult to image the medial breast.

- An inferior MLO to demonstrate the inframammary fold, the lower inner and lower outer quadrants, and the inferior portion of the upper medial quadrant (Fig. 7.14).

Depressed Sternum

Two views may again be necessary with a depressed sternum (Fig. 7.15):
- A superior MLO
- A lateral-medial of the lower quadrants

A lateral-medial is chosen because the detector plate table lies within the depression, facilitating visualization of the medial portion of the breast and the inframammary fold.

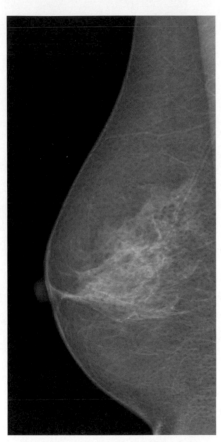

Fig. 7.14 Inferior mediolateral oblique.

Prominent Lower Ribs

Craniocaudal Projection. It is difficult to achieve a good CC in a woman with this skeletal variation. A slight rotation of the gantry by approximately 10 degrees may be beneficial. The woman should be asked to lean forward as much as possible, from the waist, but not to the extent that her head gets in the radiation field. The nipple will frequently not be in profile.

Mediolateral Oblique Projection. Rotating the gantry to between 35 and 40 degrees for the MLO will assist in positioning, by allowing the detector plate to be placed between the inframammary fold and the prominent portion of the ribs.

Variation in chest wall shape occasionally means a manual exposure is required to accomplish the required exposure factors to visualize the breast tissue.

MAMMOGRAPHY IN WOMEN WITH BREAST IMPLANTS

Efficacy of Mammography

The question of mammography on women with implants is a difficult one. Inevitably, as the implant is radioopaque, visualization of all the breast tissue is often impossible. The policy adopted for imaging women with implants should be clearly defined by a locally and/or nationally agreed protocol. Women attending for mammography should be made aware that only limited examination may be possible and that, for them, breast self-examination plays an important part in the detection of breast abnormalities. Despite the limitations, many women with implants still wish to have mammography and with improvements in digital imaging, the sensitivity of screening is increased in this group.

Anxieties of Women With Implants

The woman with implants may have additional concerns regarding mammography. Sometimes it may be difficult to recognize that a woman has implants. They may be anxious about rupturing the implants and considerable reassurance that great care will be taken, will need to be given. The risk of

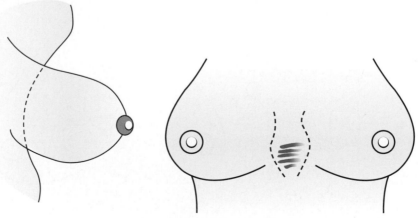

Fig. 7.15 The depressed sternum is concave in shape making it difficult to image the medial breast.

rupture of an implant as a result of performing mammography is very small. The mammographer should document in writing, with the woman's knowledge, the presence of any deformity or asymmetry of a prosthesis before performing mammography. Some services will obtain written consent to confirm the risks have been explained.

Having gained the woman's confidence, the mammographer should ascertain what proportion of the breast is formed by the prosthesis, and whether they were inserted subglandular or subpectoral because this is important in deciding which technique should be used. The greater the proportion of the breast occupied by the implant, the more difficult it is to obtain satisfactory mammograms. If more

than 75% of the breast volume is occupied by the prosthesis, mammography is likely to be of limited diagnostic value.

Positioning Techniques

Each mammography service should have a predetermined policy for the examination of women with breast implants, but in the United Kingdom, the National Health Service Breast Screening Programme has issued guidance for consistent imaging of women with breast implants. The mammographer will need to evaluate the most appropriate technique to be employed for each individual:

- Standard technique (Figs. 7.16 and 7.17)
- Eklund technique (Figs. 7.18–7.21)

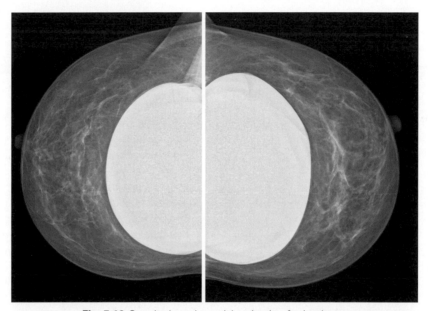

Fig. 7.16 Standard craniocaudal projection for implants.

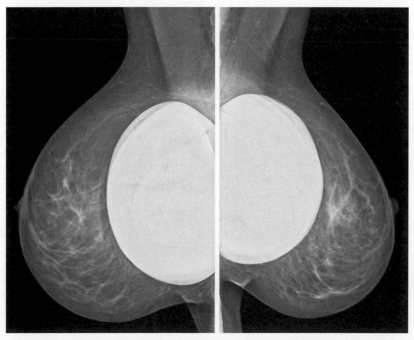

Fig. 7.17 Standard mediolateral oblique for implants.

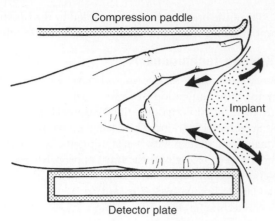

Fig. 7.18 Pull breast tissue forward from the implant.

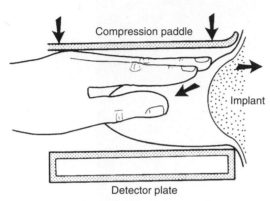

Fig. 7.19 Compression is applied to the breast tissue only.

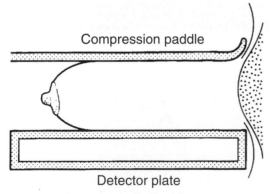

Fig. 7.20 Final position for a craniocaudal Eklund projection.

- Lateral views
- Tangential views

Craniocaudal Projections

- Exposure factors
  When applicable, the implant algorithm should be selected for postprocessing of the images. A manual exposure may have to be selected and one CC image taken initially to evaluate the exposure factors selected.
- Breast positioning
  Breast positioning is as for routine CC projection.

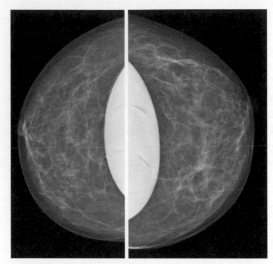

Fig. 7.21 Eklund views in the craniocaudal projections.

- Compression
  Compression should only be applied to the level at which it will hold the breast in position. Further compression will not enhance image quality, and will simply cause discomfort to the woman and heighten any anxieties with regard to rupture of the implant.
  The image should be evaluated before continuing with the rest of the examination or repeated if necessary.

Mediolateral Oblique Projections

- Exposure factors
  The exposure factors are increased by approximately one-third.
- Breast positioning
  Breast positioning is as for routine MLO projection.

Eklund Technique

Whenever possible, the Eklund technique should be employed as this is the best way to clearly visualize the natural breast tissue. This involves displacement of the implant to the back of the breast behind the compression paddle with the result that only the breast tissue is compressed and imaged. This technique is particularly successful where the implant has been placed posterior to the pectoralis major. In these cases full demonstration of the breast tissue can be achieved. This is most commonly performed in the CC projection, but an MLO projection can be used.

The procedure is as follows:
1. Palpating the anterior border of the implant, pull the breast tissue away from the implant, forward onto the detector plate (see Fig. 7.18).
2. Ease the compression paddle downwards onto the anterior breast tissue past the implant (see Fig. 7.19).
3. The anterior breast tissue is compressed and the implant pushed back toward the chest wall (see Fig. 7.20). The resultant images are shown in Fig. 7.21.

Supplementary Technique: Lateral Projection

This projection is useful if an Eklund view is not possible, most likely as a result of very scant breast tissue or an implant placed anterior to the pectoralis major (subglandular).

• Exposure factors

The exposure factors are increased by approximately one-third.

• Breast positioning

Breast positioning is as for routine lateral projection.

Supplementary Technique: Tangential Views

These can be performed in women with implants who are referred for mammography as part of the investigation of a localized lump in the breast. This is particularly useful when the implant is preventing complete evaluation of a specific area.

The procedure is as follows:

1. Palpate the "lump" or area of concern, pull the breast tissue forward onto the detector plate, away from the implant, with the "lump" in profile.
2. Ease the compression paddle downwards onto the breast past the implant.
3. The portion of the breast tissue surrounding the "lump" is compressed and the implant pushed back toward the chest wall.

MAMMOGRAPHY OF THE MALE BREAST

Although very rare, breast cancer in men does occur; therefore mammography is occasionally necessary (Fig. 7.22). The potential embarrassment of a man undergoing mammography must be recognized and the communication skills and professional manner of the mammographer in these particular circumstances cannot be overemphasized.

The standard examination consists of bilateral CC and MLO views. Positioning technique is similar to that described earlier in this chapter. Steep gantry angles and slim compression paddles can help achieve high quality images.

Practical difficulties encountered are:

• That the pectoral muscle is well developed and the breast tissue, as a general rule, is minimal. Accurate positioning, with the pectoral area not pulled excessively across the top of the film, will facilitate the application of compression.
• Hair on the chest can also mean that the compression plate tends to slide down the skin surface, but it will ultimately grip as it reaches the soft tissue of the breast itself.
• Because of the scant breast tissue, relative to the pectoral muscle it can be difficult to position the nipple. Care must be taken as this may make image interpretation difficult.

MAMMOGRAPHY OF THE POSTOPERATIVE BREAST

Surgery to the breast may be for benign pathology, cosmetic reasons, or for treatment of breast cancer. Once the breast has been subjected to surgery, there will be vastly varying degrees of deformity to the breast tissue (Figs. 7.23 and 7.24). If the woman has also had additional treatment, such as radiotherapy, there will be

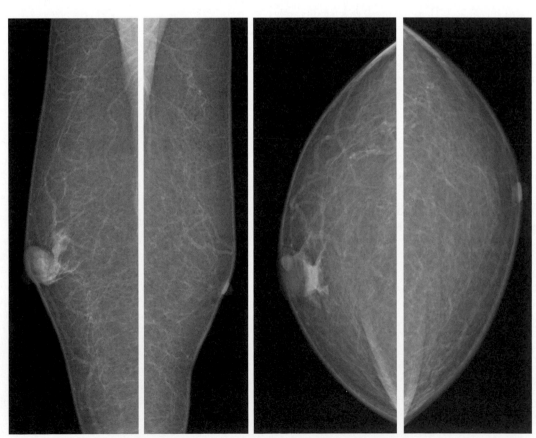

Fig. 7.22 Standard mammographic projections in a man.

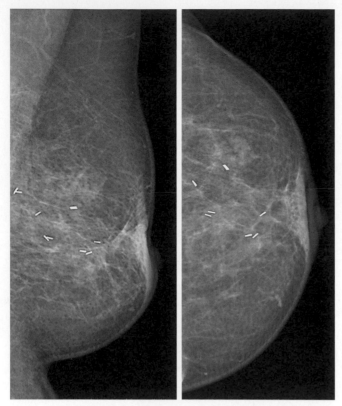

Fig. 7.23 Mammograms of a treated left breast.

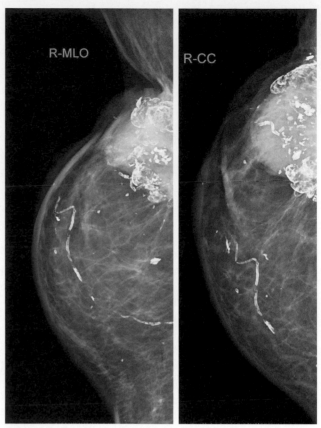

Fig. 7.24 Mammograms of a treated right breast with significant post-treatment change.

further changes to the breast. These changes may significantly increase the technical difficulty for the mammographer imaging the breast and for the woman, as long-term pain and discomfort are often associated with the post-treated breast. Multiple views may be required to demonstrate the whole breast and additional care and consideration taken when applying compression.

Extremely complex surgery is not uncommon and many women will have procedure where it is not easy to tell if there is any significant change to their breast or it is normal posttreatment change. Mammographers should be aware of their local policies for how and when to image the post-treated breast.

WOMEN WITH DISABILITIES AND/OR MENTAL HEALTH CONDITIONS

The physical and/or mental capacity of any woman may make a full or complete investigation unachievable; this may be a temporary condition or permanent.

The mammographer will have to work with the woman to ensure they are able to get the best possible mammogram for that individual at that moment in time. It is recognized that despite best efforts, optimal images are not always possible. It may also be as simple as offering an appointment at a time more suitable to their needs.

Most units have manual handling and technique training to enable the mammographer to adapt to a variety of circumstances. Sometimes it may only be possible to image a percentage of the breast tissue.

TRANSGENDER AND NONBINARY PEOPLE

The first-line investigations for transgender and nonbinary people include the standard mammography views or ultrasound, depending on the age of the individual.

It is important to maintain dignity and respect at all times and it may be necessary to arrange an appointment at the beginning or end of a clinic or in the local static unit.

FURTHER READING

Andolina, V. (2011). *Mammographic imaging: a practical guide* (3rd ed.). Philadelphia: Wolters Kluwer/Lippincott Williams & Wilkins Health.

Dumky, H., Leifland, K., Fridell, K. (2018). The art of mammography with respect to positioning and compression—A Swedish perspective. *Journal of Radiology Nursing*, 37(1), 41–48.

Eklund, G.W., Busby, R.C., Miller, S.H., Job, J.S. (1988). Improved imaging of the augmented breast. *American Journal of Roentgenology*, 151(3), 469–473.

Harvey, J., March., D.E. (2013) *Making the diagnosis: a practical guide to breast imaging*. Philidelphia: Saunders Elsevier.

Hogg, P., Kelly, J., Mercer, C. eds (2015). *Digital mammography. A holistic approach*. Switzerland: Springer International Publishing.

Huppe, A.I., Overman, K.L., Gatewood, J.B., Hill, J.D., Miller, L.C., Inciardi, M.F. (2017). Mammography positioning standards in the digital era: Is the status quo acceptable? *American Journal of Roentgenology*, 209(6), 1419–1425.

Kopans, D.B. (2006). *Breast Imaging* (3rd ed). Baltimore, Maryland: Lippincott Williams & Wilkins.

Mackenzie, A., Warren, L.M., Wallis, M.G., et al. (2016). The relationship between cancer detection in mammography and image quality measurements. *Physica Medica*, 32(4), 568–574.

Miglioretti, D.L., Rutter, C.M., Geller, B.M., et al. (2004). Effect of breast augmentation on the accuracy of mammography and cancer characteristics. *JAMA*, 291(4), 442–450.

Nightingale, J.M., Murphy, F.J., Robinson, L., Newton-Hughes, A., Hogg, P., (2015). Breast compression – An exploration of problem solving and decision-making in mammography. *Radiography*, 21(4), 364–369.

Popli, M.B., Teotia, R., Narang, M., Krishna, H. (2014). Breast positioning during mammography: Mistakes to be avoided. *Breast Cancer: Basic and Clinical Research*, 8(30), 119–124.

Public Health England. (2017). *NHS Breast Screening Programme Guidance for breast screening mammographers*. 3rd Ed. Available at: https://assets.publishing.service.gov.uk/government/uploads/system/uploads/attachment_data/file/819410/NHS_Breast_Screening_Programme_Guidance_for_mammographers_final.pdf (Accessed 20/04/20)

Public Health England. (2018). *Breast screening mammography: ergonomics good practice*. October. Available at: https://www.gov.uk/government/publications/breast-screening-ergonomics-in-screening-mammography/breast-screening-mammography-ergonomics-good-practice (Accessed 20/04/20)

Public Health England. (2019) Information for Trans and Non-Binary People. NHS Screening Programmes. Available at: https://assets.publishing.service.gov.uk/government/uploads/system/uploads/attachment_data/file/834656/Screening_for_trans_and_non-binary_people_Sept_2019.pdf (Accessed 17/04/20)

Reynolds, A., (2014). Quality assurance and ergonomics in the mammography department. *Radiologic Technology*, 86(1), 61M–79M.

Shetty, M.K. ed. (2014). *Breast cancer screening and diagnosis: a synopsis*. New York: Springer.

Shiffman, M. (2009). *Breast augmentation*. Berlin Heidelberg: Springer.

Radiologic Procedures

CHAPTER CONTENTS

OBJECTIVES

This chapter outlines:
- Why radiologic procedures are carried out
- The radiographic technical requirement of these procedures
- The types of equipment used
- The mammographers role in these procedures
- The common complications of these procedures and what actions to take

INTRODUCTION

Investigating a potential breast abnormality will usually involve one or more radiologic procedures and investigations. These are either clinically driven by the presence of a palpable and/or visible abnormality or as a result of a screening examination.

Improvements in the technical quality of mammography and widespread mammographic screening for asymptomatic women have both led to the detection of an increasing number of clinically impalpable breast abnormalities that require further radiologic workup to establish a diagnosis. The National Health Service Breast Screening Programme (NHS-BSP) publishes guidance for the assessment of screen detected abnormalities dependent on the mammographic appearances and the level of suspicion. Appearances are often subtle and care is needed by the mammographer and responsible assessor (RA) in selecting and executing appropriate complementary imaging to ensure the correct diagnosis is reached.

Whether recalled from screening or presenting symptomatically, women undergo triple assessment. This involves clinical breast examination, followed by imaging (usually mammography and/or breast ultrasound in the first instance) and histology in the form of needle sampling if necessary. The clinical and radiologic aspects are classified on a five-point risk scale advocated in the United Kingdom by the Association of Breast Surgeons and the Royal College of Radiologists' breast group:

1. Normal
2. Benign
3. Indeterminate, probably benign
4. Probably malignant
5. Malignant

The objective of investigating any breast abnormality is to reach a definitive diagnosis, with the least number of investigatory steps, in the shortest time possible and with minimum inconvenience to the woman. Imaging investigations, in conjunction with clinical breast examination, may be sufficient in some cases to enable a normal/benign diagnosis and discharge. However, there must always be concordance between the investigations resulting in a normal or benign outcome; should the clinical and radiologic assessment of suspicion be at variance then the higher degree of suspicion determines the action.

In all other cases, tissue diagnosis by needle sampling is necessary for definitive diagnosis. Image-guided core biopsy is the method advocated for sampling in the breast and either core biopsy or fine needle aspiration cytology when sampling axillary lymph nodes. The three aspects of diagnosis, clinical examination, imaging ± needle sampling make up triple assessment which is the backbone of breast investigation.

SYMPTOMATIC PRESENTATION

Reaching a definitive diagnosis can often be more straightforward in cases where the woman presents with a palpable and/or visible abnormality. Good clinical history taking is essential in helping to assess the level of suspicion and direct imaging investigations. Increased skill mix within breast clinics means this may be undertaken by one of several health care professionals trained in clinical breast examination. Historically the domain of the breast surgeon, this is now likely to be undertaken by a breast care nurse, breast physician, advanced practice radiographer, or even a radiologist. National guidance from the Association of Breast Surgeons and local protocols ensure safe and consistent practice.

In line with guidance from the Royal College of Radiologists, most symptomatic breast units undertake mammography in women aged 40 years and over. Below this threshold the often dense glandular tissue of younger women reduces mammographic sensitivity by up to 50% with a commensurate increase in dose. These women undergo ultrasound examination in the first instance with complementary mammography only if ultrasound findings are suspicious.

Digital breast tomosynthesis (DBT) can be helpful in cases of subtle mammographic change, such as asymmetry or distortion, also in assessing the extent of an abnormality especially in the dense breast. Historically, DBT has not been useful in the assessment of microcalcification but this is changing with technologic advances. DBT as a technique is discussed in Chapter 6.

SCREENING ASSESSMENT

More often than in the symptomatic setting, screen detected abnormalities are impalpable. The RA and mammographer have the joint responsibility of ensuring that all significant impalpable abnormalities are properly assessed. The RA may be a consultant radiologist, consultant radiographer, or breast clinician but must be competent in all aspects of triple assessment. Initial assessment involves confirming that an abnormality is actually present using further two-dimensional (2D) mammography and/or DBT, usually followed by breast ultrasound in the first instance. If additional 2D mammography is used, views are tailored to best demonstrate the type of abnormality being assessed. For example, workup of microcalcification must always include a lateral view to help distinguish the classic "teacup" appearances associated with fibrocystic change which in some cases can negate the need for biopsy. A magnification view is also often helpful in this. These views also assist in accurate targeting of any subsequent x-ray guided biopsy. Overall responsibility for the assessment case is taken by the RA. Good communication between RA and the mammographer working together on the case is paramount in obtaining the optimal imaging to best demonstrate the area under assessment and reach the correct outcome for the woman. NHSBSP publishes guidance on this assessment process.

Abnormalities that show characteristically benign imaging features can be safely left without further intervention. However, many have imaging features that cannot be called definitely benign and require some form of tissue diagnosis. This should be achieved by using image-guided core biopsy. There are major advantages to women, and the clinicians managing their problem, in having a reliable tissue diagnosis at an early stage. Abnormalities that are very likely to be benign can be confirmed as such and surgical intervention can be avoided. The majority of screen-detected impalpable abnormalities fall into this category. When malignancy is suspected, preoperative confirmation means that women can be provided with fully informed counseling and offered the most appropriate treatment choices; it also allows the surgeon to plan and perform surgery as a one-stage procedure, rather than diagnostic biopsy followed later by wider excision or mastectomy.

CORE BIOPSY PROCEDURES

Spring loaded automatic core biopsy devices are widely used for sampling breast abnormalities. The biopsy device takes small "cores" of tissue from the breast to be examined under the microscope. If the lesion is cancerous, a core biopsy gives diagnostic information about the tumor, including grade and type. These procedures can be performed by the RA or an advanced practitioner (the term "practitioner" will be used to encompass these professionals). The practitioner requires the assistance of a mammographer, assistant practitioner, or health care assistant. As roles are becoming increasingly blurred, the term "clinical team" will be used to describe this group in the remainder of this chapter.

IMAGE-GUIDED CORE BIOPSY

Ultrasound Guidance

For abnormalities visible on ultrasound, breast biopsy under ultrasound guidance is the procedure of choice as it is quick to perform, inexpensive, very accurate (with real-time visualization of the abnormality while it is being sampled) and, most importantly, is associated with minimal discomfort and morbidity for the woman. Core biopsy is advocated for sampling the breast while fine needle aspiration cytology is also acceptable when needle sampling axillary nodes.

For abnormalities not visible on ultrasound, such as microcalcification, x-ray guided biopsy is usually performed. Fig. 8.1 shows the simple decision-making process.

X-Ray Guidance

For all abnormalities not visible on ultrasound and not definitely benign, x-ray guided sampling is necessary. This is commonly known as a stereotactic-guided biopsy.

It is important that mammographers have a full understanding of why and how localization of impalpable breast abnormalities are performed as they play an integral part in the process; practitioners rely on the expertise and skill of mammographers for the procedure to be successful.

Significant mammographic lesion

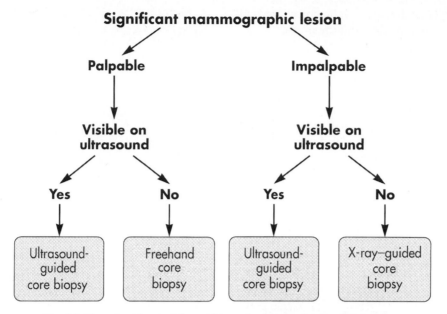

Palpable → Visible on ultrasound → Yes → Ultrasound-guided core biopsy

Palpable → Visible on ultrasound → No → Freehand core biopsy

Impalpable → Visible on ultrasound → Yes → Ultrasound-guided core biopsy

Impalpable → Visible on ultrasound → No → X-ray–guided core biopsy

Fig. 8.1 Flow chart for deciding which method to use for needle sampling.

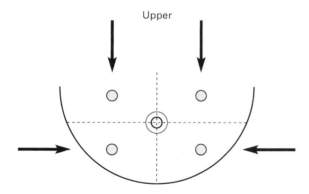

Upper

Fig. 8.2 Approach for localization according to breast quadrant. Choose the shortest route between skin entry point and lesion as possible. For example: approach from above (CC position) if lesion is in the upper breast or from the lateral aspect if the lesion is in the lower outer quadrant.

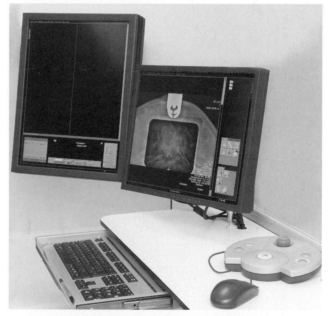

Fig. 8.3 Acquisition monitor for stereotactic procedures.

The positioning skills of the mammographer are challenged by increasingly subtle findings following the introduction of digital mammography. Consideration should be given to the position of the lesion in the breast (Fig. 8.2); if the lesion is positioned too high or low in the breast, the equipment will not allow targeting to happen. This is for the safety of the woman and to protect the detector plate. Modern equipment allows the procedure to be adapted to different approaches to optimize tissue sampling and comfort.

The Mammography Room

The size and design of the room to be used for x-ray guided procedures are important. The room chosen will need to be larger than a standard mammography room and should have sufficient space to accommodate with ease the mammography equipment and its accessories, the woman, and clinical team, but should not be so large that the woman feels vulnerable and exposed. Storage cupboards for biopsy and localization items should be in the room so their contents are quickly and easily available. The room should be maintained at a temperature in which the woman will feel neither too hot nor too cold; optimal ambience is best achieved with an efficient air conditioning system. It is very important to ensure that the room temperature does not rise too high as this will increase the likelihood of the woman fainting during the procedure and the equipment overheating. The clinical team should be fully involved in the design and planning of any new mammography facility.

As interventional procedures are performed with digital mammography, the images can be viewed on the acquisition monitor to help plan the procedure and to select and localize the area of concern (Fig. 8.3). Mammographers should familiarize themselves with how to target for stereotactic procedures and how to select the appropriate needle from the menu.

The Equipment

Stereotactic-guided interventional breast procedures can be performed within existing upright mammography equipment (Fig. 8.4) with add-on features or specially purchased specially designed prone biopsy tables or biopsy chairs (Fig. 8.5). Cost and available space plays a major part in which system is available. DBT is now available for use in clinical practice to perform interventional procedures under image guidance.

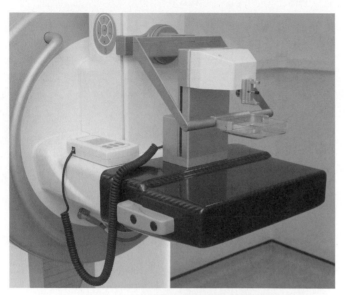

Fig. 8.4 Conventional stereotactic biopsy unit.

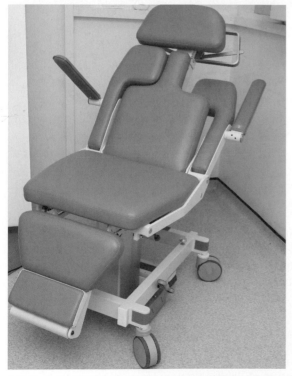

Fig. 8.5 Dedicated biopsy chair for use with upright or decubitus localization procedures.

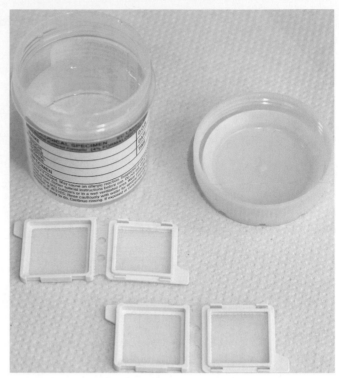

Fig. 8.6 Specimen containers for needle core biopsies.

Once they have been obtained, the biopsy samples will be sent to histopathology for analysis in specimen sample pot containing formulin to preserve the sample (Fig. 8.6).

Preliminary Imaging

The clinical team must work together to decide which complementary views will demonstrate the location of the abnormality within the breast, to accurately target any subsequent biopsy.

As already discussed, lateral views and magnification paddle views help characterize microcalcification and assess extent (see Chapter 6). Depending on the location of the abnormality in the breast, complementary views, such as an extended craniocaudal (CC), may help visualize an abnormality in the axillary tail (see Chapter 6). Sometimes an abnormality, such as distortion, may be seen in only one projection; targeting for biopsy must then be performed using this projection. It is the mammographer, and not the practitioner, who has the difficult task of positioning the woman correctly for the procedure. In addition to the location in the breast, some physical conditions, such as cervical spondylosis or frozen shoulder, may preclude use of standard positions. In these circumstances the true lateral approach is often successful and is likely to be best tolerated.

The Intervention

Before any intervention is undertaken, particularly x-ray guided procedures which are more complex and require a compliant woman, the procedure must be explained simply and fully to the woman. The woman is much more likely to consent to the procedure and cooperate if she has been informed of both why and how the test is performed. The success of image-guided procedures is often directly related to the skill and experience of the operators. Explanation is reassuring and helps to establish good rapport between the woman and the clinical team. The ambience should be relaxed, with the woman aware and confident that the procedure is routine to the team carrying it out. The woman can be engaged in conversation as much as required throughout with regular reminders of what is about to happen and frequent updates on how much longer the procedure is going to take.

The shortest possible needle route to the lesion should be considered and x-ray guided procedures can be undertaken with the woman sitting (Fig. 8.7) or lying in the prone or decubitus position (Fig. 8.8). The latter are facilitated by either a dedicated prone table or biopsy chair with the

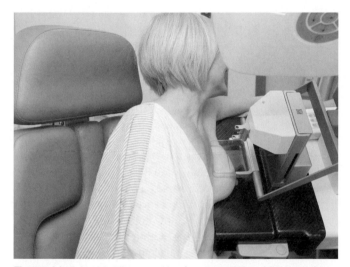

Fig. 8.7 Mediolateral oblique position for stereotactic-guided procedures.

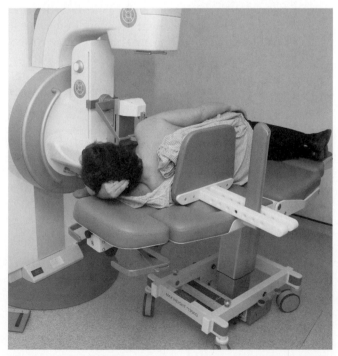

Fig. 8.8 Lateral decubitus position for stereotactic-guided procedures.

capacity to recline, as shown in Fig. 8.5, which require specific positioning techniques.

There is anecdotal evidence the woman is less likely to suffer light-headedness or faint during or after the procedure if she is lying. However, some locations in the breast would best be targeted with the woman in the upright position if this is the shortest distance for the biopsy needle to traverse the breast. The clinical team must agree to the approach, taking into account the likely compliance of the individual woman. This can be assessed during preprocedure consultation, as described earlier.

The number of staff involved in any one procedure should be kept to a minimum. Ideally, there should be up to three: the practitioner, the mammographer, and an assistant to look after the woman. Women do not appreciate too many staff being around unless they know who everyone is and why they are there. If trainees are involved, the woman should be asked in advance if they mind them being present to observe; very few will object if asked politely. The woman must never be left unattended and should be supervised until the practitioner has confirmed that the procedure has been completed and that the woman is fit to leave the department. An examination couch with a head-down tilt facility should be available to lie the woman down, should she experience light-headedness or faint during or after the procedure (see complications later).

Tips for the Mammographer

The role of the mammographer cannot be overemphasized. Some key factors need to be observed in all stereotactic procedures:

- It is helpful if the mammographer has had contact with the woman before; rapport will have already been established and the mammographer will be familiar with the site of the lesion.
- A woman's comfort is paramount if the procedure is to be successfully completed.
- If the woman is seated, this should be in a suitable chair with the lower lumbar area fully supported throughout the procedure so that the woman is not tempted to move.
- The lesion should be located as quickly and accurately as possible. This will minimize discomfort, unnecessary exposures, and possible movement or syncope.
- Having positioned the woman, the outline of the "window" in the compression plate can be marked on the skin so that any subsequent movement of the breast will be evident.
- The woman should not be left alone while the procedure is underway.
- The mammographer should empathize with and support the woman throughout the procedure.

The Procedure for Stereotactic Localization

The mammographer should fully understand the technique of stereotactic localization. The principles described are applicable to all stereotactic localization procedures. The mammographer should:

1. Check that the equipment and materials are correctly assembled before the woman arrives.

2. Explain the method and purpose of the radiographic processes to the woman as they are performed. Using upright equipment, the risk of the woman fainting during the procedure is considerably reduced if the woman is reassured and relaxed.

3. Position the woman and apply the compression paddle after agreeing the ideal breast position with the practitioner (Fig. 8.9). It is important to get accurate positioning for an optimal procedure, but is also imperative that the woman is able to tolerate compression throughout. It is worthwhile spending some time involving the woman in the process to get her full cooperation.

4. A marker pen should be used to draw the outline of the compression paddle window on the skin (Fig. 8.10).

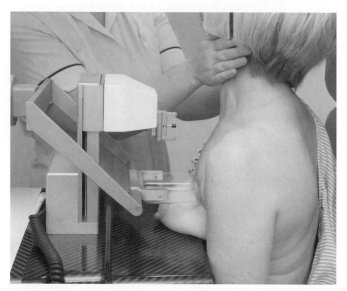

Fig. 8.9 Positioning for a craniocaudal procedure.

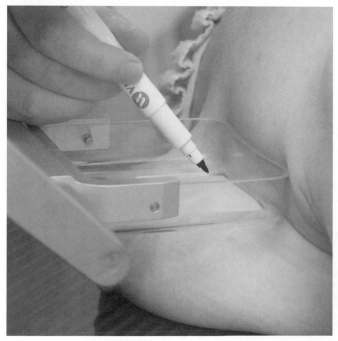

Fig. 8.10 Marking the boundaries.

Movement of the breast under the compression paddle during the procedure will then be easy to detect.

5. Carry out the x-ray tube movements required to obtain the stereo images. For upright systems, it is often necessary to place the woman's head in an awkward and uncomfortable position (see Fig. 8.9) when the x-ray tube is being rotated. Care is required to avoid movement of the breast under the compression paddle—the pen marks on the breast should be checked to ensure that their relationship to the compression plate window has not changed (see Fig. 8.10).

6. The scout view will be shown on the acquisition monitor. Check the scout projection to make sure the area of interest is included in the field of view, within the aperture of the compression paddle and will not be projected off the images when the stereotactic projections are taken (Fig. 8.11). If the area is not clearly visible, the woman has moved, or is too close to the edge of the compression paddle, the woman should be repositioned before proceeding and a repeat scout view taken.

7. If the area of concern is well placed in the aperture proceed to the stereotactic pair (Fig. 8.12).

8. Check the stereotactic images with the practitioner. The woman should be repositioned if the abnormality is not clearly demonstrated or it is close to the margin of the compression paddle edge. It is better to reposition the woman than accept a suboptimal position for most cases; on rare occasions a compromise is necessary but may result in an overall suboptimal procedure.

9. Once satisfactory stereotactic images are obtained, the lesion will be targeted to calculate the coordinates. For the depth calculation to be accurate, it is essential that exactly the same part of the abnormality is visible and selected on both the stereotactic images and that the reference point has been accurately marked. If the same point cannot be targeted either movement of the breast may have occurred or the area of concern may be too close to the detector plate or the skin surface. Repositioning of the woman will be required. The method of calculating coordinates using the stereotactic images

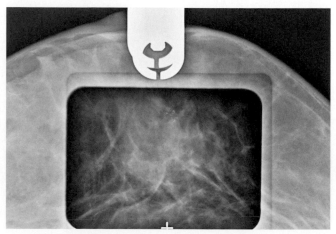

Fig. 8.11 Scout view demonstrating the area of concern.

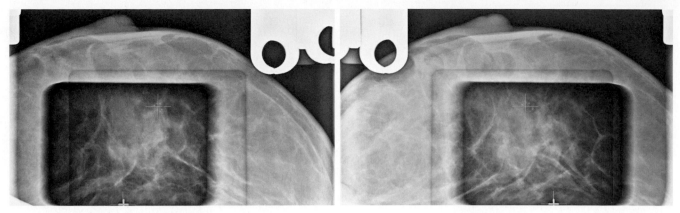

Fig. 8.12 Stereotactic pair with the area of concern targeted for sampling.

varies considerably according to the make and model of the equipment. This part of the procedure is not described here.

10. Once accurate coordinates have been calculated, the biopsy system will move the needle guides to the area of concern; the needle can be placed in the guides so that it is directly above the targeted area (Fig. 8.13).

11. Local anesthesia is administered, a small incision is made, and the needle is placed in the breast.

12. In some units, it is standard practice to take check images to confirm that the needle is in the correct position.

13. Multiple passes may be made for each procedure to ensure the area of concern is fully sampled.

VACUUM-ASSISTED PROCEDURES

Vacuum-assisted biopsy (VAB) is another method, which takes samples on tissue, using a variety of gauge needle, by "sucking" tissue into the needle. It can be used under ultrasound or x-ray guidance.

The type and position of the lesion in the breast will determine the approach used. This is for the safety of the woman and to protect the detector plate. Modern equipment allows the procedure to be adapted to different approaches to optimize tissue sampling and the woman's comfort but because of the size of vacuum devices, this is currently much more limited. The increased amount of tissue obtained is more likely to give detailed and accurate information about the lesion targeted than the traditional core biopsy, but there are limitations, such as risk of bleeding and hematoma formation, more expensive equipment, and increased time required for reporting by the pathologist.

For VABs, the lateral approach in conjunction with a lateral arm probe holder offers some advantages to upright systems compared with the vertical approach (Fig. 8.14). The lateral approach allows for accurate biopsy in smaller breasts where the compressed depth may be too small to allow for vertical biopsy. This technique also facilitates easier access to the retroareolar area and close to the chest wall. Fig. 8.15 shows the principle of VAB.

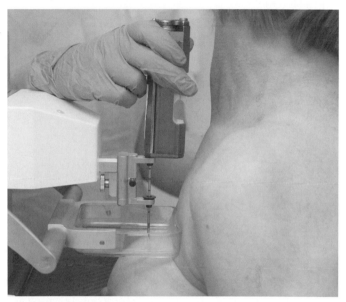

Fig. 8.13 The area is targeted and the biopsy needle in the correct position ready to take a sample.

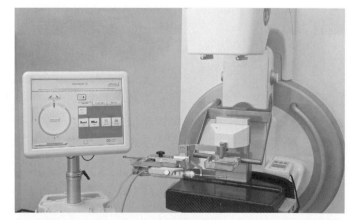

Fig. 8.14 Setup for lateral approach vacuum-assisted biopsy with specially adapted lateral arm attachment.

Whereas 14-gauge core biopsy is the traditional method, when available stereotactic VAB is advocated for sampling microcalcification, as the vacuum assistance and larger bore needle allows more extensive sampling and a greater likelihood of reaching a definitive diagnosis. Some units use VAB

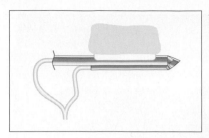

1 Stereotactic or ultrasound guidance used to position the probe

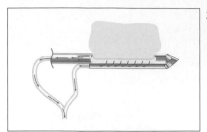

2 Tissue is gently vacuum aspirated into the aperture

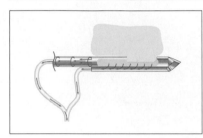

3 The rotating cutter is advanced, cutting and capturing a specimen

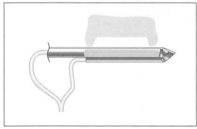

4 After the cutter has reached its full forward position, rotation and vacuum cease

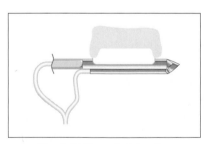

5 The cutter is withdrawn transporting the specimen to the tissue collection chamber while the outer probe remains in the breast

Fig. 8.15 The principle of vacuum-assisted biopsy.

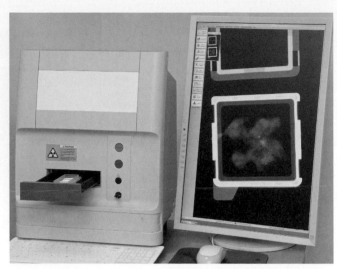

Fig. 8.16 Dedicated specimen cabinet for imaging biopsy samples.

for all x-ray guided sampling while others may use core biopsy in the first instance.

Since the use of VAB equipment has become more widespread, some lesions which are indeterminate (of uncertain malignant potential) on core biopsy can undergo vacuum-assisted excision (VAE) rather than surgical removal. If the abnormality is amenable (not too close to skin or pectoral muscle), this can be done under ultrasound guidance using the same equipment as for a VAB, this time hand held by the operator. Alternatively, this can be done under x-ray guidance. Optimal VAE sampling yields 4 g of tissue as advocated by the NHSBSP. There is also published guidance as to which lesions are amenable to vacuum excision and which, because of their increased malignant potential, require surgical excision.

SPECIMEN IMAGING

Core biopsy and vacuum samples are large enough to allow the samples to be x-rayed. This is useful when the area of concern has microcalcification involved, as x-raying the specimens can confirm or exclude the presence of representative calcification within the specimens. This can increase the confidence level that the correct area has been targeted for sampling or may result in additional samples being taken; it is a valuable and speedy practice giving almost instant feedback on the success of the procedure.

Specimen radiography of biopsy samples can be performed with magnification on a conventional mammography machine, but the use of a specimen cabinet is currently the most widely used option (Fig. 8.16).

IMAGE-GUIDED LOCALIZATION WITH TISSUE MARKERS AND WIRES

Mammography screening and improved mammography equipment mean more small cancers are diagnosed with core biopsy. These are often impalpable and their location in the breast can be marked at biopsy by a clip which is made of titanium and inert, but visible on mammography (Figs. 8. 17 and 8. 18).

There are various shapes available. It is prudent to keep several in the department as sometimes more than one clip is deployed to mark multiple areas of abnormality and it is important to be able to distinguish between them. Indeterminate areas requiring surgical excision can be clipped in a similar way at biopsy and in all such cases, localization can then be undertaken under ultrasound guidance, which like core biopsy is the simplest method. When no clip is visible on mammography, either no clip was placed/clip failed to deploy, migration has occurred or it is not included in the field of view.

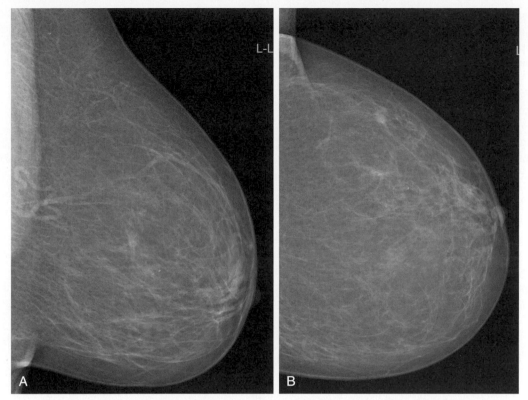

Fig. 8.17 Small impalpable screen detected lesion in the left breast in the (A) lateral and (B) craniocaudal projections.

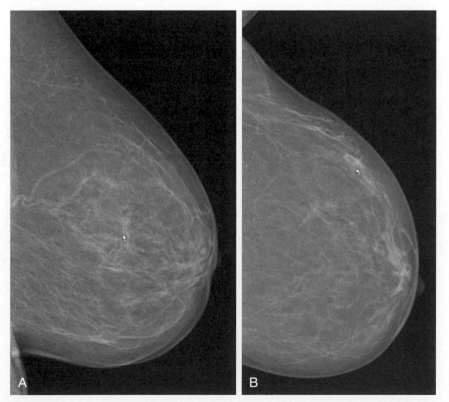

Fig. 8.18 Postbiopsy mammograms showing tissue marker at the site of the targeted lesion in the (A) lateral and (B) CC projections.

Women undergoing neoadjuvant chemotherapy may also have a marker clip placed, so that in the event of complete radiological response, the tumor site can still be localized.

When the management of an impalpable lesion is surgical excision, image-guided localization is required. This may be under ultrasound or x-ray guidance, and are mostly likely to involve the placement of either a wire (Fig. 8.19) or magnetic seeds.

The lesion and/or marker clip are identified as they would be for core biopsy, local anesthetic is administered, and a preloaded cannulated needle is used to introduce the wire or magnetic seeds. Postprocedure CC and lateral mammograms are obtained to demonstrate the location of the targeted area within the breast. Once the wire is inserted, postprocedural images are taken to demonstrate the proximity of the wire to the targeted area (Fig. 8.20).

Surgically excised localized specimens will be imaged (Fig. 8.21), usually with a specimen cabinet in theatre or in the mammogram machine to ensure the targeted lesion has been excised, with apparent disease-free margins.

COMPLICATIONS

The risk of introducing infection through carrying out image-guided procedures is minimal. However, these procedures should be carried out using aseptic technique. Gloves should be worn for the protection of the woman and staff. The mammographic or ultrasound equipment used must be thoroughly cleaned with bactericidal solution before and

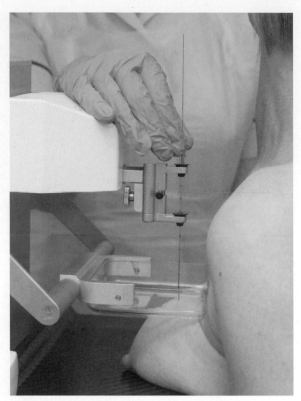

Fig. 8.19 Preparing for a wire-guided localization under stereotactic guidance.

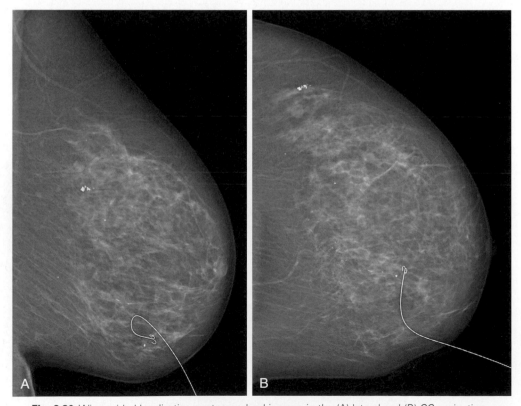

Fig. 8.20 Wire-guided localization postprocedural images in the (A) lateral and (B) CC projections.

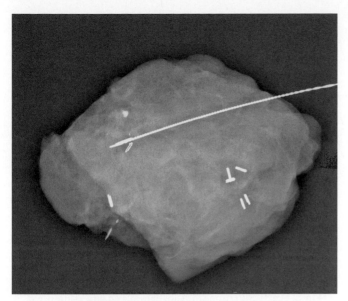

Fig. 8.21 Postsurgical specimen x-ray.

after each woman to ensure that the small risk of cross-contamination with blood is eliminated. Advice on which solutions can be safely used on equipment is usually provided by the manufacturers, if not the hospital sterile supplies department or control of infection officer will give advice. It is preferable for all biopsy devices to be single use; where this is not possible, it should be sterilized as per hospital policy.

Complications are uncommon and are less likely to happen when the team performing the procedures is experienced in the techniques. It is the practitioner's responsibility to ensure that the procedure to be performed is adequately explained to the woman and to ensure that there are no contraindications, such as anticoagulant therapy and allergy to local anesthetic.

Pain and Tenderness

Most of the pain associated with any needling procedure is caused by the puncturing of the skin, where the pain nerve endings are concentrated. This is usually limited to immediate sharp pain felt as the needle passes through the skin. Local anesthetic should be used to anesthetize the skin for biopsy where the needle gauge will require a skin nick with a scalpel blade but the merits of its use must be decided for other procedures. If only a single fine-bore needle is going to be used, for example, for cyst aspiration, then local anesthesia is probably not necessary, as the injection of the anesthetic agent may be more painful than the procedure itself. The pain associated with injection of local anesthetic can be reduced by warming the anesthetic fluid to body temperature before it is injected.

Bleeding and Bruising

Slight bleeding occurs with virtually all needling procedures and is exacerbated by the hyperemia and venous congestion caused by the compression of the breast used in the various x-ray techniques. About half of women will develop a visible bruise at the site of needle puncture that will resolve over the next 5 to 7 days. Bruising is often accompanied by mild localized tenderness that subsides quickly and can be relieved by mild oral analgesia if necessary. To avoid unnecessary anxiety, women should be warned that bruising and tenderness are likely to develop. Usually, Steri-Strips and a simple skin dressing is applied to the puncture site (nonallergenic dressing for women with allergy to adhesive plasters). This is to protect the women's clothing from blood staining and to reduce the risk of infection. She can be advised to remove the dressing in the next 24 hours (this may vary according to local protocol).

Bleeding may be more pronounced after a VAB and firm pressure should be applied to the puncture site and above the biopsy tract postprocedure, using the flat of the hand, for at least 10 minutes or until bleeding stops. Bleeding can be minimized by using local anesthetic combined with adrenaline. Significant bleeding is rare but can occur if a small blood vessel is inadvertently transfixed. Should significant bleeding occur during the procedure, it should be suspended until the bleeding stops. Occasionally, a procedure will need to be completely abandoned because of bleeding. A pressure bandage can be applied but is rarely necessary.

Safety and Blood Spillage

As in any situation where some bleeding is inevitable, all medical personnel likely to have direct contact should take all necessary precautions and wear protective gloves, preferably latex free. Care should be taken when cleaning and clearing away any items and areas where there has been blood spillage. All mammographers should be fully aware of and practice their unit's policy and guidelines on handling blood and blood-stained equipment. All equipment that is not disposable must be thoroughly cleaned and sterilized after each woman. Cleaning and sterilizing solutions should be compatible with the equipment—check the manufacturers' instructions. Every mammography assessment center should have its own guidelines for these cleaning procedures.

Light-Headedness and Syncope

Light-headedness is relatively uncommon, occurring in less than 3% of women in our experience, and is more likely when the room is humid and the temperature too high. Women who complain of light-headedness during any procedure should be asked to breathe slowly and deeply through the mouth. Most episodes can be relieved by this maneuver with progression to fainting avoided and the procedure completed successfully. Ask the woman if they have experienced light-headedness or fainting during previous, similar procedures. If so, they are more likely to have similar problems again and it is wise to observe them closely. Engage them in conversation to distract attention throughout the procedure. Any woman who has experienced light-headedness should be asked to lie down for a short while afterwards until the RA or practitioner is happy that they have fully recovered.

In a small number of women, light-headedness will progress to fainting (syncope). These women must be closely observed and the procedure abandoned at the first sign of fainting. In these circumstances, lie the woman down in the recovery position with her head placed lower than the body and legs. Most women recover consciousness very quickly and should be offered ample reassurance as they do so. They should be encouraged to remain lying for at least 15 minutes. Again, women should only be allowed to leave after being checked over by the RA/practitioner.

FURTHER READING

Aminololama-Shakeri, S., Soo, M.S., Grimm, L.J., et al. (2019). Radiologist-patient communication: current practices and barriers to communication in breast imaging. *Journal of the American College of Radiology*, 16(5), 709–716.

Andolina, V. (2011). *Mammographic imaging: a practical guide* (3rd ed.). Philadelphia: Wolters Kluwer/Lippincott Williams & Wilkins Health.

Barkhausen, J., Rody, A., Schafer. F.K.W. (2016). *Digital breast tomosynthesis: technique and cases*. New York: Thieme.

Borrelli, C., Cohen, S., Duncan, A., et al (2016). NHSBSP; Clinical guidance for breast cancer screening assessment, publication 49. Public Health England. Available at: https://associationofbreast-surgery.org.uk/media/1414/nhs-bsp-clinical-guidance-for-breast-cancer-screening-assessment.pdf (Accessed 20/04/20)

Ganott, M., Griffith, B., Rudzinski, S.M. (2019). Breast imaging and image-guided biopsy techniques. *Breast Disease*, 63–94.

Giess, C.S., Frost, E.P., Birdwell, R.L. (2012). Difficulties and errors in diagnosis of breast neoplasms. *Seminars in Ultrasound, CT and MRI*, 33(4).

Harvey, J., March, D.E. (2013). *Making the diagnosis: a practical guide to breast imaging*. Philidelphia: Saunders Elsevier.

Hogg, P., Kelly, J., Mercer, C. eds (2015). *Digital mammography. A holistic approach*. Switzerland: Springer International Publishing.

Johnson, K., Sarma, D., Hwang, E.S. (2015). Lobular breast cancer series: imaging. *Breast Cancer Research*, 17(1).

Kopans, D.B. (2006). *Breast imaging* (3rd ed). Baltimore, Maryland: Lippincott Williams & Wilkins.

Kuzmiak. C. ed (2019) *Interventional Breast Procedures: A Practical Approach*. Springer International Publishing. Available at: DOI 10.1007/978-3-030-13402-0

IAEA (2012). *The Critical Examination of X-Ray Generating Equipment in Diagnostic Radiology*. Medical Engineering and Physics (MEP). Available at: https://www.ipem.ac.uk/ScientificJournalsPublications/TheCriticalExaminationofX-RayGeneratingEquip.aspx

Nori, J., Kaur, M. (2018). *Contrast-enhanced digital mammography (CEDM)*. Springer International.

Perry, N., Broeders, M., de Wolf, C., Törnberg, S., Holland, R., von Karsa, L. (2008). European guidelines for quality assurance in breast cancer screening and diagnosis. —summary document. *Annals of Oncology*, 19(4), 614–622.

The Royal College of Radiologists. (2019). *Guidance on screening and symptomatic breast imaging 4th edition*. November. Clinical Radiology. Available at: https://www.rcr.ac.uk/system/files/publication/field_publication_files/bfcr199-guidance-on-screening-and-symptomatic-breast-imaging.pdf (Accessed 20/04/20).

Shetty, M.K. ed (2014) *Breast cancer screening and diagnosis: a synopsis*. New York: Springer.

Wagner, J., Liston, B., Miller, J. (2011). Developing interprofessional communication skills. *Teaching and Learning in Nursing*, 6(3), 97–101.

Training, Education, and Continuing Professional Development in Mammography Practice

OBJECTIVES

This chapter outlines:
- Training and education requirements for radiographers
- Specialist education for radiographers in mammography
- Role development opportunities

INTRODUCTION

From the early 1990s the national rollout of the National Health Service Breast Screening Programme (NHSBSP) saw state registered radiographers taking up mammography posts in breast imaging. They underwent additional training to achieve the required competency in providing mammography services. The subsequent evolution of initial radiography training from diploma to a graduate framework heralded consolidation of the additional mammography training as the postgraduate Certificate of Competence in Mammography awarded by the Society and College of Radiographers (SCoR). This involves 1 year's Masters level training requiring radiographers to have not only in-depth knowledge of mammography and mammographic services, but also the ability to research best practice in both mammography and the wider diagnostic service. State-registered radiographers in mammography not only provide a high-quality clinical mammography service but are also enquiring and proactive practitioners who can influence the service from an evidence base.

At the time of writing, there is evidence of a continued historical shortage of both radiographers qualified as mammographers and radiologists in the United Kingdom. There is an ever-increasing demand for mammography services and this demand is expected to continue to rise as a result of demographic increases, heightened breast awareness among the population and retirement of the first cohorts of radiographers and radiologists trained in breast imaging.

WORKFORCE PRESSURES

The increased workload and ever-reducing staff numbers will create tremendous pressures on the diagnostic service. Unless an additional workforce is identified to address the increased service, diagnosis will be delayed. This will also create barriers to role development at a time when the opportunity has finally arrived to move beyond the traditional boundaries of radiography.

The recent revisions to the Ionizing Radiation (Medical Exposures) Regulations (IR[ME]R) provide opportunities for state-registered radiographers to take greater responsibility and accountability within the service. These regulations also allow the use of nonstate-registered practitioners working under the supervision of a state-registered practitioner. The nonstate-registered practitioners will have to be suitably trained and have competence assessed. This review of the rules governing irradiating patients has led to the development of a potential additional radiographic workforce.

Assistant/Associate Mammography Practitioners

The role of assistant practitioner was a remodeling of radiographic working introduced in the early 2000s to address the first signs of staff shortages, including a shortage of radiographers trained as mammographers. Training routes for assistant practitioners have evolved with time and are currently being consolidated into a mammography associate apprenticeship involving 1 year's clinical and academic training. Assistant practitioners and mammography associates can undertake specific mammography examinations as directed by their scope of practice and will work under the supervision of state-registered radiographers. The scope of practice for these roles is evolving in light of the continued shortages in the United Kingdom radiographic workforce.

Expanding the Role of the Postgraduate Mammographer

Some of the radiographic workforce have continued their postgraduate studies to become advanced practitioners by adding usually clinically based modules, such as mammography reporting and breast ultrasound to their portfolio. This role progression is vital for sustainability in the radiology crisis also being experienced across the United Kingdom. The current academic criteria expected by the SCoR for an advanced practitioner is a full Master's degree. There are various routes to achieving this and other less clinical modules, such as family history/genetics counselling or health promotion can be added depending on local need. An advanced practitioner may continue to develop further to achieve the relevant skills, competencies and academic requirements of a consultant role. For both advanced and consultant practitioners, there is an expectation to undertake four pillars of practice; in addition to demonstrating expert clinical practice should undertake research, professional leadership, and teaching. Consultant practitioners work autonomously and have the capability to take on many of the actions traditionally performed by a radiologist, as a result, professional boundaries have become blurred.

AUDITING MAMMOGRAPHIC CLINICAL PRACTICE

For an autonomous profession, auditing clinical practice is essential. Each mammographer needs to review and reflect on clinical practice as part of regular personal performance monitoring. Continued monitoring of mammographic skills will help to maintain and improve the quality of service provided to clients. Attaining and maintaining high-level clinical skills will not occur without the continued pursuit of excellence. To facilitate audit of personal performance, all images are electronically annotated with a personal identifier.

REVIEW OF REPEATED EXAMINATIONS

One method is to review technical recall and technical repeat (TR/TP) rates. The percentage of repeat examinations should be as low as possible. This is important so that radiation dose is kept to a minimum and that repeat images do not raise anxiety and potentially deter women from subsequent attendance for breast screening.

Repeat images can provide evidence of both equipment issues and mammographer performance. Regular monitoring will provide opportunities for remedial action in both areas. If the technical recall rate is caused by equipment malfunction,

the frequency of this should be noted and the equipment taken out of service if images are likely to be undiagnostic.

In the case of repeat images resulting from the technical skills of the mammographer performing the examination, reviewing the work will identify trends in practice and identify any further training needs. Film reader preference may also influence TR/TP rates and will require auditing.

MAMMOGRAPHIC IMAGE QUALITY ASSESSMENT

In 1993 performance criteria and a grading system for mammographic practice were introduced and incorporated into the training syllabus and the quality assurance guidelines for mammography. This was commonly called the "PGMI system" where images were graded as perfect, good, moderate, or inadequate. The implementation of this system was met with some apprehension but over time it was implemented throughout the United Kingdom both for training and ongoing performance monitoring. This system was also widely adopted by Australia, New Zealand, and Hong Kong. The great strengths and benefits of this system were that a clear standard for mammography clinical practice was established and that the constant striving to achieve films in the "perfect" and "good" categories had a marked effect in raising the quality of mammography. Another strength of the system was that radiographers reviewed a whole series of examinations from both their own clinical practice and that of their mammography colleagues on a regular basis. This enabled informal comparisons to be made, discussions to take place, and practice to be influenced.

However there were limitations in the PGMI system; research indicated that the scoring was subjective and that different individual practitioners produced different scores on the same sets of images. This made individual, unit, or regional comparisons difficult. In addition, analogue imaging was replaced by digital mammography. There was discussion around mammographers having to make subtle changes in their positioning largely because of digital equipment being more bulky to work with. There seemed to be an adaptation of positioning, including more variation of angle (usually flatter than the proposed value of 45 degrees with PGMI).

In 2017, the previous NHS breast screening guidance of 2007 was replaced by a revised image assessment tool. This is still current and the mandatory method within the screening program for image review. It is an integral part of assessment during training and as an ongoing process at individual, peer, and department level. It is recommended that a mammographer should audit at least 20 mammograms every 2 months, following specific criteria. A summary of the criteria found in the tool can be found in Table 9.1

With the advent of digital mammography, real-time image review is now widely available. This enables any repeats to be undertaken at the time of examination without necessitating recall for the client. In addition, software on departmental workstations allows retrospective review of individual and team performance with indicators for trends in positioning error and areas for further training.

REVIEWING MAMMOGRAMS

Scrutinizing a mammographic examination and comparing left and right projections can help in identifying positioning errors. This technique relies heavily on the understanding of the mammographer relating what is happening to the breast and the body while positioning takes place and how compression affects the breast tissue. This skill takes some time to develop, but once gained, turns a competent mammographer into an expert one. Common quality factors for discussion in all examinations are:

- absence of movement
- adequate compression
- correct annotations
- correct exposure
- correct digital processing
- absence of artefacts
- symmetrical images
- nipples in profile
- skin fold free
- whole breast imaged

  Others topics of discussion relate to the specific projection (Table 9.1). For example, discussions about technique factors in the craniocaudal (CC) projection could be:
- evidence of pectoral muscle at the back of the film
- position of the pectoral muscle if evident
- relationship between the posterior nipple line and the back of the image
- demonstration of medial and lateral borders
- depth of the breast tissue from nipple to back of the image

  For the mediolateral oblique (MLO) projection, discussions would include:
- height of the machine
- relationship between the length of the pectoral muscle and the level of the nipple
- the angle of the pectoral muscle
- demonstration and openness of inframammary angle

EXAMPLES OF MAMMOGRAMS FOR IMAGE REVIEW

Examples of mammographic examinations, image grading, and discussion points relating to positioning factors can be found below (Figs. 9.1–9.12).

Craniocaudal Mammograms

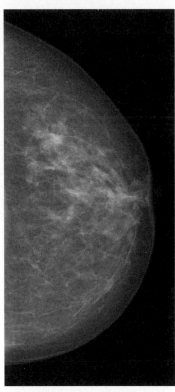

Fig. 9.1 A perfectly positioned craniocaudal projection. The nipple is central and the posterior nipple line is at 90 degrees to the back of the image. Pectoral muscle is subtly visible at the back of the image. There is good visualization of the medial and lateral breast with the nipple in profile.

TABLE 9.1 Summary of Criteria for Assessing Mammograms	
Summary of Criteria for Assessing Mediolateral Oblique Images	**Summary of Criteria for Assessing Craniocaudal Images**
• correct patient identification (ID) and markers • appropriate exposure • adequate compression to hold breast firmly—no movement • image sharp • no artefacts obscuring image • no obscuring skin folds • nipple in profile (should normally be demonstrated in at least 1 view) • pectoral muscle to nipple level (or posterior nipple line) • pectoral muscle at appropriate angle • inframammary angle shown clearly • symmetrical images • whole breast imaged	• correct patient ID and markers • appropriate exposure • adequate compression to hold breast firmly—no movement • image sharp • no artefacts obscuring image • no obscuring skin folds • nipple in profile (should normally be demonstrated in at least 1 view) • medial border demonstrated • back of breast clearly shown with some medial, central, and lateral • some axillary tail shown • symmetrical images • whole breast imaged

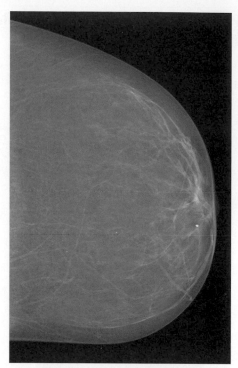

Fig. 9.2 An adequately positioned craniocaudal projection. The pectoral muscle is just visible so the back of the breast is included but the breast is slightly medially rotated and the nipple is not in profile.

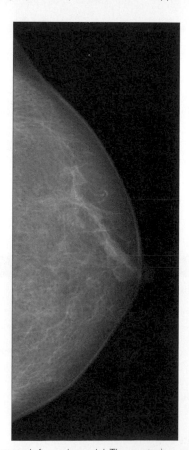

Fig. 9.3 Inadequate left craniocaudal. The posterior part of the breast is not included; glandular tissue is transected at the back. The breast is medially rotated, so the nipple is not central and possible loss of medial breast tissue.

Mediolateral Oblique Mammograms

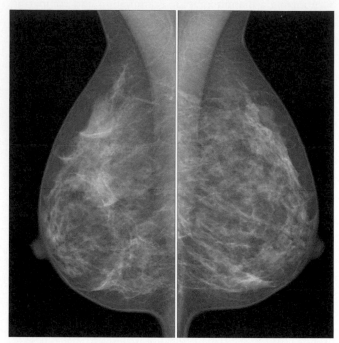

Fig. 9.4 Perfect mediolateral oblique images. The breasts are symmetrical. The pectoral muscle is very evident down to nipple level. The inframammary angles are also visible both confirming the breast has been pulled forward adequately and all of the breast tissue is visible. The nipples are in profile.

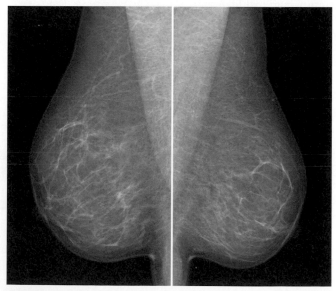

Fig. 9.5 Very good mediolateral oblique mammogram. The breasts are almost symmetrical, but the left is slightly more angled than the right breast. This is likely caused by a difference in where the woman was standing in relation to the detector plate for each view. The pectoral muscle is very evident down to nipple level. The inframammary angles are also visible both confirming the breast has been pulled forward adequately and all of the breast tissue is visible. The nipples are in profile.

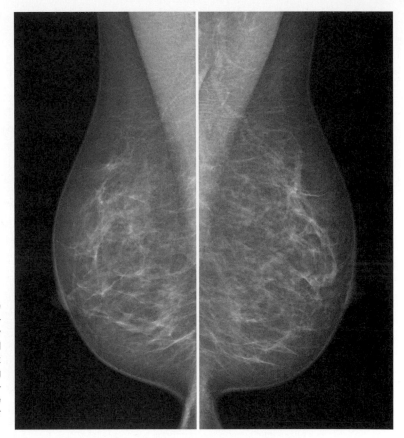

Fig. 9.6 Good mediolateral oblique mammogram. Slight nipple rotation bilaterally; the woman may have her hips slightly rotated or the breast tissue has not been pulled through fully from the back. The muscle is not quite down to nipple level and is not quite symmetrical. There is a small skin fold at the back of the left pectoral muscle and small folds are also beginning in the inframammary area. There is more volume of breast tissue on the left than right; this may be caused by a difference in size of the breasts, it is essential the mammographer records this when performing the mammogram.

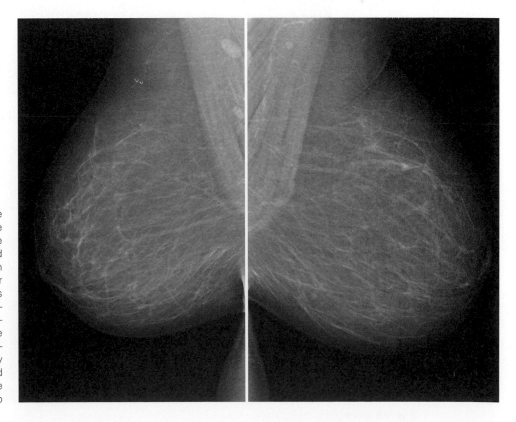

Fig. 9.7 Adequate mediolateral oblique mammogram. There is a crease in the upper part of the left breast. The muscle is not symmetrical; this is likely caused by a difference in where the woman was standing in relation to the detector plate for each view. There are skin folds at the back of both breasts, more evident on the left. The inframammary angles are untidy and tissue could be missed; this may be caused by the angle the woman is leaning into the x-ray machine. She may need to stand straighter and tuck her bottom in. The height of the detector plate may need to be adjusted.

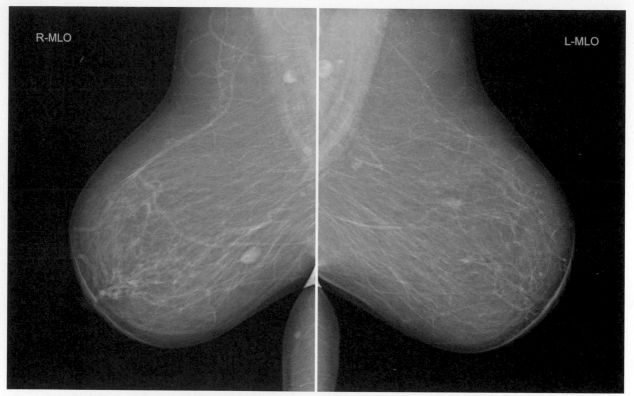

R-MLO

L-MLO

Fig. 9.8 Adequate mediolateral oblique mammograms. The breasts have not been lifted sufficiently. This makes them sag and the inframammary angles are not visualized, with small skin folds. There is possible loss of breast tissue in the posterior and lower breast.

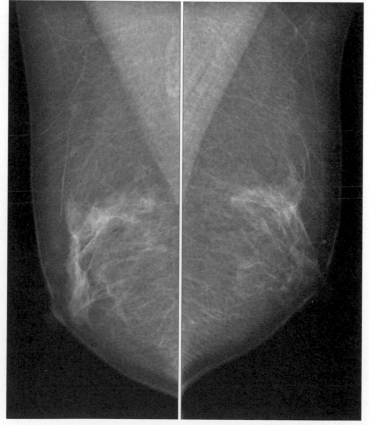

Fig. 9.9 Inadequate mediolateral oblique mammograms. The breasts are not lifted, the nipples are down-turned, and the inframammary angles are not visible. There is definite loss of breast tissue.

Complete Mammogram Examination

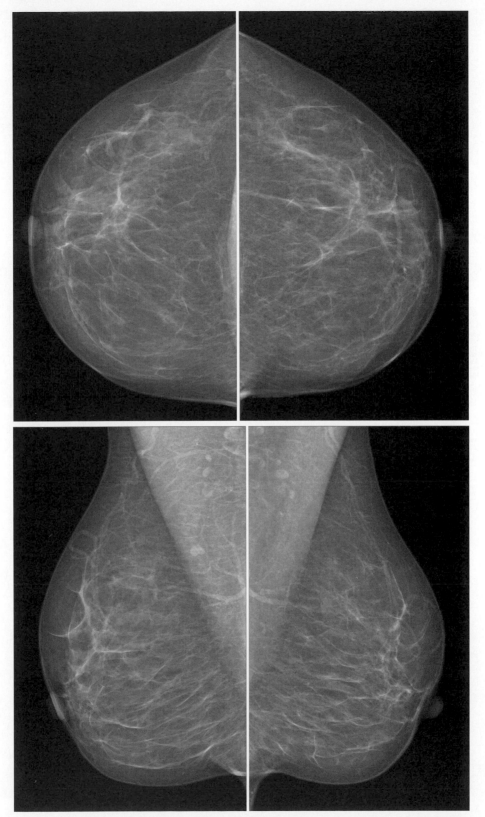

Fig. 9.10 Good mammogram. The images are symmetrical. The muscle is down to the level of the nipple. The muscle is at an appropriate angle. The right nipple is slightly turned and there are small creases in the inframammary area which is more prominent on the right but these do not obscure much tissue. A good quality craniocaudal view will help to ensure all of the tissue is seen clearly. The medial and lateral edges are demonstrated on the images. The pectoral muscle can be seen on the right side but not on the left. Both nipples are very slightly out of profile. The images are all sharp with no blurring.

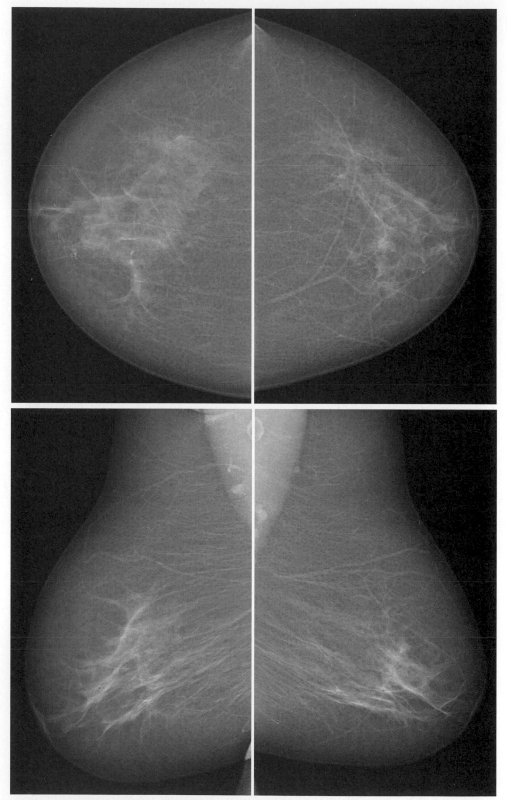

Fig. 9.11 Adequate mammogram. The nipples are in profile on all four views. The muscle is not down to the level of the nipple on either side for the mediolateral oblique views. There is a fold in the right inframammary angle and the left may be missing. On the craniocaudal views the muscle cannot be seen on either side but following the 1 cm rule, the same volume of tissue is demonstrated as the mediolateral oblique views. This may be a woman with physical challenges and supplementary views as described in Chapters 6 and 7 may be required.

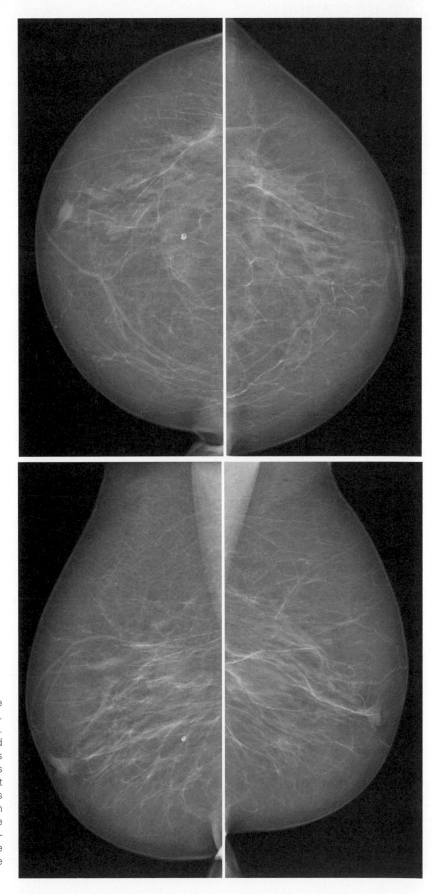

Fig. 9.12 Inadequate mammogram. Mediolateral oblique projections—the nipple is not in profile on either side. There is very little muscle demonstrated on either side. In addition, the angle of the muscle is very steep and it is not down to the nipple. The inframammary fold is untidy on both sides.Craniocaudal view—the nipple is not in profile on the right side. The pectoral muscle is not seen on either breast and using the 1 cm rule, there is less tissue on both craniocaudal views compared with the mediolateral oblique views. These problems may be caused by the physical condition of the woman and supplementary views as described in Chapter 6 should be considered, such as nipple views, to fully image the breast.

FURTHER READING

Andolina, V., Lille, S. (2011). *Mammographic imaging: a practical guide* (3rd ed.). Philadelphia: Wolters Kluwer/Lippincott Williams & Wilkins Health.

Hogg, P., Kelly, J., Mercer, C. eds (2015). *Digital mammography. A holistic approach.* Switzerland: Springer International Publishing.

Jasper, M. (2013). *Beginning reflective practice.* (2nd ed). Andover: Cengage Learning.

Kopans, D.B. (2006). *Breast Imaging* (3rd ed). Baltimore, Maryland: Lippincott Williams & Wilkins.

Moran, S., Warren-Forward, H. (2011). A retrospective study of the performance of radiographers in interpreting screening mammograms. *Radiography*, 17(2), 126–131.

Nass, S.J., Patlak, M. (2015). Assessing and improving the interpretation of breast images. In Nass, S.J., Patlak, M. eds. *Assessing and improving the interpretation of breast images* (1st ed.). National Academies Press.

Perry, N., Broeders, M., de Wolf, C., Törnberg, S., Holland, R., von Karsa, L., (2008). European guidelines for quality assurance in breast cancer screening and diagnosis. —summary document. *Annals of Oncology*, 19(4), 614–622.

Public Health England. (2017). *NHS Breast Screening Programme Guidance for breast screening mammographers.* 3rd Ed. Available at: https://assets.publishing.service.gov.uk/government/uploads/system/uploads/attachment_data/file/819410/NHS_Breast_Screening_Programme_Guidance_for_mammographers_final.pdf (Accessed 20/04/20)

Tabar, L., Dean, P., Boulter, P. (2012). *Teaching atlas of mammography.* (4th ed). Stuttgart, Germany: Thieme Publishing Group.

Théberge, I., Guertin, M.-H., Vandal, N., et al. (2018). Clinical image quality and sensitivity in an organized mammography screening program. *Canadian Association of Radiologists Journal*, 69(1), 16–23.

Quality Assurance Systems

OBJECTIVES

This chapter outlines:
- The coordination of quality assurance processes into a comprehensive system
- The key points to look for in a quality assurance program

- Organizational requirements for a quality service internal and external quality assurance system
- Differing types of mammographic services with different objectives

INTRODUCTION

The effectiveness of a mammography service depends upon the outcomes and can be judged by measuring performance against stated objectives. The performance of the service as a whole is dependent on how well each of its constituent parts performs.

QUALITY ASSURANCE

Quality assurance (QA) is a way of maintaining and improving the quality of service delivery and outcomes by paying attention to every part of the process through systematic review and monitoring. It is a way of minimizing mistakes and making the service cost efficient and effective. From beginning to end all aspects of breast care services are connected and influence each other to ultimately impact on patient outcomes. An error in any part of the proceeding may not result in a catastrophic event but it makes for a safer patient journey if there are multiple opportunities for errors to be detected and rectified.

Assuming no process is perfect, there is opportunity for error at every point. A good quality assurance system will detect weaknesses at each stage and put processes into place to detect any errors, if they do not meet the correct criteria to pass through to the next stage. The effectiveness of processes and outcomes will be established by the continuous monitoring and feedback associated with a comprehensive quality assurance program.

Developing a Quality System

There are a variety of models used in business that have been adapted for use in health care such as Total Quality Management (TQM) and the (Lean) Six Sigma strategy. All models outline a structured approach to process mapping, gathering data, maintaining standards, and implementing improvements; they work from the ground up breaking down quality processes designed for individual elements, building to create the overall high quality service delivery.

A QA system is made up of several separate elements:
- the definition of objective,
- the identification of criteria, whereby the objectives may be measured,
- the agreement of standards,
- the collection of information,
- the review of performance,
- following the review, the definition of new objectives, the confirmation of the validity of criteria, and the introduction of new criteria is required. Similarly standards should be changed if they prove to be too lax or too ambitious.

Definition of Objectives

Defining clear quality objectives of any service, maps out the expectations and commitment to provide safe, high-quality care for both participants and service users. Quality objectives may be related to processes or outcomes from the overall service and through each individual element involved in the client journey.

The overall outcome objective for a breast screening service could be defined as the reduction in mortality from breast cancer in the targeted population. Each section of the service could define several different objectives relating to differing roles in the screening process, for example:

- a mammographer to produce excellent mammograms
- a reader to detect the maximum number of small cancers
- the surgeon to achieve a low incidence of cancer recurrence

These are process objectives, and each of these has its own quality cycle.

Identification of Criteria

Criteria must be simple, meaningful, and repeatable. They should represent exactly what is being measured. Importantly, they should be easily understood and easily implemented. Examples of criteria relating to process objectives defined for the UK National Health Service Breast Screening Programme (NHSBSP) are given in Table 10.1.

Agreement of Standards

To recognize the good and bad in any process or outcome, the standards must be measurable and be audited.

There are two types of standards: those that are acceptable and those that are achievable. Acceptable standards represent the minimum performance required to achieve the objectives to which they relate. Achievable standards represent the level of performance that the service should aspire to. These are standards achieved by the best 10% of services, and are of value as targets for units which are performing less well. Standards of both types should be agreed by the profession to which they relate. Examples of both acceptable and achievable standards are given in Table 10.1. The NHSBSP QA program is the culmination of a series of evidence-based quality processes that guide and monitor all aspects of service delivery and outcomes. As the program has evolved, new and improved standards have been developed and implemented to cover all aspects of service delivery; an example can be seen in Table 10.2.

Collection of Information

The key to an accurate and efficient quality assurance process is the availability of accurate data, without which it is impossible to monitor performance. The UK NHSBSP collects data through a national database system which collates and analyzes the data in an efficient and meaningful way. Essentially the same objectives, and therefore criteria and standards, can be adopted by units providing services for symptomatic women. The data required to monitor the effectiveness and efficiency of a symptomatic breast imaging service are very similar to those needed for the quality assurance system of a screening service.

Review of Performance

It is important that a review of performance is a productive process and perceived as an opportunity to learn. It should be conducted on the basis of nonjudgmental, open discussions, aimed at motivating in areas of underperformance,

and congratulating in areas of achievement. In addition to group reviews, it is of great importance that individuals should review their own performance, measuring this against the approved standards and the performance of their peers (personal performance audit).

Organizational Requirements

The NHSBSP has an established set of standards and criteria against which services, professions, and individuals are measured to ensure a safe high-quality service to clients. Over the years, a series of multidisciplinary publications have been developed to guide and quantify the expectations of service providers and service users. These are regularly updated in light of new evidence. However, each individual service is required to have their own governance and supporting documentation demonstrating how they apply the criteria into their everyday practice to meet the national standards. In order that the various elements within a mammographic service can function to the best possible standards, it is essential that the optimal organizational environment is provided within which they can function efficiently.

Culture and Education

A culture of learning and reflection will help promote motivated conscientious practitioners. Poor technique and limited knowledge can lead to a poor experience for the women and possible misdiagnosis. All staff must be fully trained in the techniques they are using and must maintain and improve their knowledge through continued professional development, reflection, and audit.

Availability and Accessibility

In the public eye, the quality of a service depends on an appreciation of the reasonableness of any restrictions placed upon the woman who might attend, and the geographic accessibility of the service to that woman.

When restrictions are in force, such as age limitations for a screening service, the reasons for these should be clearly stated to the general public. Women who request a service, but are refused, should be given details of any appropriate existing alternatives which may be available. Should a woman complain of a breast problem and request an appointment at a unit which is not geared to providing the type of service she really requires, it is an essential of good practice to advise her of the action she should take, and whom she should consult.

Geographic accessibility is a major consideration, particularly in the organization of a screening service, when maximum participation is a prime objective. Local transport availability should be considered during the determination of the siting of a service. It may be preferable to serve some areas using basic mammographic apparatus installed in a mobile caravan or trailer.

Availability of Assessment

It is essential that both basic and sophisticated mammographic services have rapid and easy access to an expert

TABLE 10.1 Examples of Criteria and Objectives for the UK National Health Service Breast Screening Programme

Standard Number	Objective	Criteria	Acceptable Standard	Achievable Standard
1 Coverage: eligible population identified and invited	To maximize timely attendance within 36 months of screening in the eligible population	The proportion of women eligible for screening who have had a test with a recorded result at least once in the previous 36 months	≥70%	≥80%
4 Test and minimizing harm: repeat examination rate	To minimize the number of women undergoing repeat examinations to minimize anxiety and exposure to radiation	The proportion of repeat examinations (because of technical recalls or technical repeats) by service (also recommended by practitioner)	<3%	<2%
5 Minimizing harm: recording appropriate radiation dose	To limit the amount of radiation dose to the glandular tissues of the breast from mammograms	Mean glandular dose (MGD) per view for a standard breast in clinical settings	≤2.5 mGy	
6 Minimizing harm and diagnosis: image quality	To maximize the numbers of cancers detected	Threshold gold thickness measured using the test object	See below	

THRESHOLD GOLD THICKNESS (µm)[a]

Diameter of Detail (mm)	Minimum Acceptable Value	Achievable Value
1	≤0.091	≤0.056
0.5	≤0.150	≤0.103
0.25	≤0.352	≤0.244
0.1	≤1.68	≤1.10

[a]Lower values of threshold gold thickness indicate better image quality

Standard Number	Objective	Criteria	Acceptable Standard	Achievable Standard
8 Minimizing harm: referral to assessment rates	To minimize the number of women screened who are referred for further tests, while trying to minimize false negative rates	The proportion of eligible women with a technically adequate screen who are referred for assessment	<10% (prevalent screen) <7% (incident screen)	<7% (prevalent screen), <5% (incident screen)
14 Diagnose: age standardized detection ratios (SDRs) for invasive cancers	To maximize the numbers of invasive cancers detected	The SDR is the ratio of the observed number of invasive cancers to the expected number in the eligible population invited and screened	1.00	1.40
18 Outcomes: rates of interval cancers	To minimize the number of interval cancers presenting between screening episodes	The number of interval cancers per 1000 women screened	<0.65/1000 diagnosed <12 months of the previous screen <1.40/1000 diagnosed between 12 and <24 months of the previous screen <1.65/1000 diagnosed between 24 and <36 months of the previous screen	Not applicable

TABLE 10.2	Example of Standards for the UK National Health Service Breast Screening Programme
Breast Screening Program Standard 11	**Minimizing Harm: Number of Assessment Visits to Obtain a Definitive Diagnosis**
Rationale	It is important to reduce anxiety in women by aiming to minimize the number of assessment visits required to obtain a definitive diagnosis. An early nonoperative diagnosis of malignancy is highly desirable as it allows informed pretreatment counselling of the patient and facilitates one-stage treatment thus ensuring that anxiety is minimized.
Objective	The number of diagnostic assessment visits needed to achieve a definitive outcome should be as low as possible.
Criteria	The minimum standard is that 95% of women should require no more than three separate visits for diagnostic assessment (including visits to receive results). The number of visits will depend on the structure of the assessment process; however no more than two needle biopsy procedures carried out on separate occasions should normally be needed to achieve a nonoperative diagnosis.
Definitions	Numerator: number of women with three or more visits for diagnostic assessment and results appointments
	Denominator: number of eligible women attending assessment
	(Both within defined period expressed as a percentage)
Performance thresholds	Acceptable: ≥95%
Mitigations	In some circumstances, repeated visits may be necessary where difficult to diagnose lesions are found to be multifocal or the multidisciplinary team (MDT) requires further investigations to be undertaken
	Some services may not have the resources to allow all investigations to be undertaken in one visit. This may lead to more than two visits for further diagnostic tests on occasion.
Reporting	Reporting focus: screening service
	Data source: National Breast Screening System
	Responsible for submission: screening service
	Annually as part of the Association of Breast Surgery audit

assessment service. In the United Kingdom, most services provide rapid access breast clinics where women will undergo a triple assessment of physical examination, imaging, and biopsy if necessary.

Professional Organization for Quality Assurance

Each professional group should undertake the establishment and operation of its own QA system. This entails the definition of professional objectives, the identification of criteria whereby they can be measured, and the setting of standards. Probably the most important part of the quality cycle to be undertaken by members of a profession is the monitoring of professional performance. Not only is a profession in the best position to understand the specifics of its own practice but members of that profession are more likely to respond to the knowledge of peers.

Internal Quality Assurance Systems

QA procedures should be adapted to reflect the resources and setup of the individual unit. There should be personal involvement of individuals working in the service, giving an appreciation of their own part in the production of a quality service. There should be routine systematic review of existing procedures to identify and change those which are suboptimal, mechanisms for reporting system failures, and necessary corrective action plans. Individual professions are also required to undertake self-audit of their personal performance and to participate in continuing professional development pertinent to their practice.

External Quality Assurance Systems

In addition to self-assessment, which is crucial to a satisfactory quality of performance, there should be a method to have performance assessed by an outside agency—an external quality assessment procedure. Radiographers and assistant practitioners in the United Kingdom have organized an accreditation system for themselves, based essentially upon a full training course with periods of attachment to an active training unit.

Similarly, readers have access to a series of test images and pathologists a series of microscope slides which are circulated to participating personnel.

There are also regular service reviews which interrogate and peer review every aspect of the service. Thus services and individuals are able to compare performance data with their peers.

THE NATIONAL HEALTH SERVICE BREAST SCREENING SERVICE QUALITY ASSURANCE SYSTEM

The NHSBSP screening quality assurance service (SQAS) is responsible for the QA of all programs up to the end of the screening pathway. Further treatment and ongoing services are governed by the relevant professional bodies and their respective standards but work closely with SQAS. Breast screening QA starts with the identification of eligible women up to the point of diagnosis, when a breast cancer is confirmed or the woman is returned to routine screening cycle.

The QA provision is led by the national team linking with the regional and local services to support the development of standardization of processes and procedures. In England, there are currently four regional quality assurance service (RQAS) teams who monitor how services meet standards and support their improvement as well as contribute to the national program.

Clinical and professional advisors share expertise and knowledge to improve quality across the program. As a group of experts they contribute to QA visits, act as national leads, and support the development of new and improved standards. All aspects of the service will have their own professional representatives.

RQAS continually assess the services within their region and help with the collation and analysis of data relating to all aspects of the service, challenging the submitted evidence in relation to quality, offering support and potential noncompliance. On occasion, a service may identify an adverse incident that may bring into question overall quality or patient safety; RQAS will support the management and resolution. They undertake regular assessments and visits to services, including peer review.

There is a full series of NHSBSP publications, produced by Public Health England, for use by various professional groups, which detail the QA processes to be adopted by each profession.

The NHSBSP has produced a systematic management program for use in all screening services. This has many of the features of the International Standard.

FURTHER READING

Andolina, V., Lille, S. (2011). *Mammographic imaging: a practical guide* (3rd ed.). Philadelphia: Wolters Kluwer/Lippincott Williams & Wilkins Health.

De Jonge, V., Sint Nicolaas, J., Van Leerdam, M.E., Kuipers, E.J. (2011). Overview of the quality assurance movement in health care. *Best Practice and Research: Clinical Gastroenterology*, 25(3), 337–347.

Department of Health. (2013). *Public health functions to be exercised by NHS England Service specification No.24 Breast Screening Programme.* Available at: www.nationalarchives.gov.uk/doc/open-government-licence/ (Accessed 17/04/20)

Hogg, P., Kelly, J., Mercer, C. eds (2015). *Digital mammography. A holistic approach.* Switzerland: Springer International Publishing.

Jones, E. (2018). Practical steps to improving the quality of care and services using NICE guidance. *NICE Website*, 1–22. Available at: https://intopractice.nice.org.uk/practical-steps-improving-quality-of-care-services-using-nice-guidance/index.html accessed 17/4/20 (Accessed 17/04/20).

Kopans, D.B. (2006). *Breast Imaging* (3rd ed). Baltimore, Maryland: Lippincott Williams & Wilkins.

National Academies of Sciences, Engineering, and Medicine. (2015). *Assessing and Improving the Interpretation of Breast Images: Workshop Summary.* Washington, DC: The National Academies Press. https://doi.org/10.17226/21805.

NHS Cancer Screening Programmes (2013) *Routine quality control tests for full-field digital mammography systems. Equipment report 1303: fourth edition* October. Available at: https://assets.publishing.service.gov.uk/government/uploads/system/uploads/attachment_data/file/442720/nhsbsp-equipment-report-1303.pdf (Accessed 16/04/2020).

Perry, N., Puthaar, E., Broeders, M., Törnberg, S., Holland, R., Wolf, C. de, Karsa, L. von. (2008). European guidelines for quality assurance in breast cancer screening and diagnosis. Fourth Edition – summary document. *Annals of Oncology*, 19(4), 614–622.

Public Health England. (2017). NHS Breast Screening Programme Guidance for breast screening mammographers. 3rd Ed. Available at: https://assets.publishing.service.gov.uk/government/uploads/system/uploads/attachment_data/file/819410/NHS_Breast_Screening_Programme_Guidance_for_mammographers_final.pdf (Accessed 16/04/20).

Public Health England. (2019). *Breast screening: guidelines for medical physics services.* Breast Screening: Quality Assurance for Medical Physics Services. Available at: https://www.gov.uk/government/publications/breast-screening-quality-assurance-for-medical-physics-services/breast-screening-guidelines-for-medical-physics-services (Accessed 16/04/2020).

Reis, C., Pascoal, A., Sakellaris, T., Koutalonis, M. (2013). Quality assurance and quality control in mammography: A review of available guidance worldwide. *Insights into Imaging*, 4(5), 539–553.

Reynolds, A., (2014). Quality assurance and ergonomics in the mammography department. *Radiologic Technology*, 86(1), 61M–79M.

Sauven, P., Bishop, H., Patnick, J., Walton, J., Wheeler, E., Lawrence, G. (2003). The National Health Service Breast Screening Programme and British Association of Surgical Oncology audit of quality assurance in breast screening 1996-2001. *British Journal of Surgery*, 90(1), 82–87.

Wilson, R., Liston, J. (eds) (2011). *Quality Assurance Guidelines for Breast Cancer Screening Radiology.* 59. Sheffield: NHS Cancer Screening Programmes. Available at: https://assets.publishing.service.gov.uk/government/uploads/system/uploads/attachment_data/file/764452/Quality_assurance_guidelines_for_breast_cancer_screening_radiology_updated_Dec_2018.pdf (Accessed 20/04/20).

The Basis of Mammographic Interpretation

CHAPTER CONTENTS

OBJECTIVES

This chapter outlines:
- The role of mammography in breast cancer diagnosis
- Common variants of normal
- Histologic types of breast cancer

- The likelihood of radiographic signs being caused by benign or malignant disease: mass lesions, spiculate lesions' architectural distortion, calcifications

INTRODUCTION

This chapter describes common abnormalities that affect the breast. An understanding of the mammographic features of breast conditions will help the radiographer to perform good-quality mammograms.

THE ROLE OF MAMMOGRAPHY

The role of mammography varies according to the reason for a woman's examination. In the breast cancer screening setting, mammography aims to demonstrate any abnormality before the woman becomes aware of symptoms. Mammography is also part of the assessment process for women referred to the breast unit, usually from their general practitioner (GP), with breast signs/symptoms. In all instances, mammography is used to exclude or confirm a malignant process. When employed in conjunction with clinical assessment and histopathology, a definitive diagnosis of benign disease may be obtained and the woman saved unnecessary surgical intervention.

It is important for the mammographer to be mindful of the setting she is in when performing the examination as this may affect the behavior of the woman or the technique necessary to optimally demonstrate the possible abnormality. Good communication will also help in assessing the woman's level of anxiety and ascertaining the nature of any presenting symptoms. Mammographers have rightly been described as crucial to the woman's pathway in being the link between the woman and the reader. Whatever the setting, observations conveyed, either by documentation during the screening episode or by conversation during handover of the woman in a symptomatic clinic, can be invaluable in correctly tailoring the next part of the woman's journey. If the assessor is forewarned of a known benign breast problem, this may help to avoid unnecessary biopsy later.

There are only a few localized benign problems that can be diagnosed with certainty on mammography. Ultrasound (US) of the breast is a useful adjunct to mammography in these circumstances, with differentiation of cystic from solid lesions and characterization of solid lesions being of particular clinical value.

The role of mammography in the assessment of malignant disease of the breast is more complex and better defined. Mammography will demonstrate the majority of palpable breast tumors and will almost always show signs helpful in differentiating benign from malignant processes. Screening mammography may also detect malignancy well before it is the cause of clinical signs or symptoms, and also as an additional incidental finding during symptomatic assessment, hence its effectiveness as a screening tool. However, not all breast cancers, even when clearly palpable, are visible on mammography. There are a variety of reasons for this. Some breasts are very dense on mammography, to such an extent that even large lesions are not discernible within the dense normal tissues. In other cases, the breast cancer is of a type that does not disrupt or disturb the normal breast architecture and hence is invisible on mammography.

Imaging plays a fundamental role in the diagnosis and treatment of breast cancer, as there is usually excellent correlation with histopathology findings. Mammography is more accurate than palpation in assessing the size of a tumor, it can show the extent of the disease by detecting multifocal disease, may show associated ductal carcinoma in situ, and will confirm that the opposite breast is disease-free. Knowledge of all these factors is essential to the proper management of breast cancer.

Indications for Mammography

Mammography is rarely indicated in young women. Almost all breast symptoms in young women are caused by benign or physiologic processes and mammography has little to offer in their management. Breast cancer is very rare under the age of 30 years. Although the incidence increases with age, evidence suggests the increase becomes more significant from the age of 40 years and cancers below the age of 40 years are more effectively diagnosed with US, which is the imaging technique of first choice in this age group. In addition, the young breast is inclined to be denser on mammography and lesions are less likely to be visible. The young breast is theoretically more susceptible to the carcinogenic effects of ionizing radiation, although the risks of cancer induction by mammography are small at any age. These factors mean that mammography is rarely indicated in the assessment of symptoms in women under 40 years of age, unless there is a strong clinical suspicion of malignancy and current guidelines support this. In the absence of symptoms, mammography cannot be justified as a screening tool in women under the age of 40 years. Mammographic screening is of proven value in women aged 40 to 70 years. The main reason for few programs screening women aged 40 to 49 years is poor cost effectiveness. Women under 50 years with a strong family history of breast cancer can be referred to the genetics department for assessment of their risk. Dependent on the results, the woman may be eligible for increased screening at a younger age with mammography and/or magnetic resonance imaging (MRI).

US should be the imaging technique of choice in younger women and is useful in the further assessment of lesions demonstrated on mammography. US is not an effective technique for screening for breast cancer at any age.

The Influence of Age and Hormone Replacement Therapy on Mammographic Sensitivity

The density of the breast on mammography does vary with age, with younger premenopausal women more likely to show a dense background pattern.

In very dense background breast patterns, the sensitivity of mammography can be reduced by as much as 50%. It is therefore not surprising that breast cancers are not always visible on a mammogram, even when clinically palpable, and that this is more likely to be the case in younger women. Hormone replacement therapy (HRT) causes an increase in mammographic density in many women and can be the cause of denser breasts in women of screening age. The Breast Imaging Reporting and Data System (BIRADS) is widely used to score mammographic density, particularly in North America and Europe and more recently in the United Kingdom. This enables consistency of practice and sharing of data between countries. BIRADS classification uses four categories from A (almost entirely fatty) through to D (very dense) commensurate with increasing density (Fig. 11.1).

MAMMOGRAPHIC FEATURES WHICH INDICATE AN ABNORMALITY

No mammographic feature can indicate that a particular lesion is benign or malignant with certainty. Some features may be highly suggestive of a benign diagnosis whereas others are typical of malignancy. However, many mammographic signs are less clear cut and the differentiation of benign and malignant conditions requires further imaging, clinical assessment, and cytologic/histologic examinations.

There are four primary mammographic features that may indicate the presence of a breast abnormality:

- Mass
- Parenchymal deformity
- Asymmetric density
- Microcalcifications

Mass

A mass is defined as a central area of increased density with generally convex margins. Masses can be divided into those that are well-defined, ill-defined, or spiculate (Table 11.1).

A well-defined mass (Fig 11.2), particularly if it shows a "halo" on mammography, is very likely to be benign whatever its size. Age is an important factor in the differential diagnosis of a well-defined mass. Under the age of 35 years, a fibroadenoma is the most likely diagnosis. Between 35 and 55 years, cysts are very common. After 55 years, the vast majority of well-defined masses are still benign but a well circumscribed

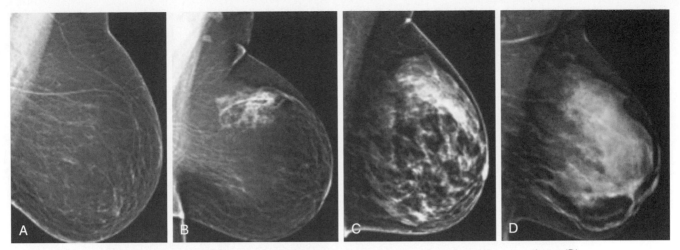

Fig. 11.1 Illustration of the variety of background breast density from very fatty (A) to very dense (D).

TABLE 11.1 Differential Diagnosis of Masses Demonstrated on Mammography

Well-Defined Mass	Ill-Defined Mass	Spiculate Mass
Cyst	Carcinoma	Carcinoma
Fibroadenoma	Hematoma	Complex sclerosing lesion
Lymph node	Fat-necrosis	Surgical scar
Papilloma	Abscess	
Abscess	Fibroadenoma	
Hematoma		
Hamartoma		

carcinoma becomes a credible possibility. Lobulation is suggestive of benignity.

Masses which appear ill-defined (Figs. 11.3 and 11.4) in any part of their margin on mammography must be considered suspicious and always require further assessment. US is ideal for distinguishing cysts from solid lesions. US is also useful in differentiating benign from malignant masses. Malignant masses on US are usually heterogeneous, poorly defined masses with distal shadowing which are often taller than they are wide (Fig. 11.5). US is also useful in defining the extent of malignant lesions.

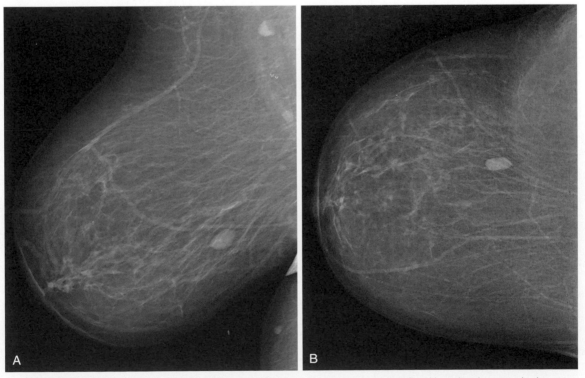

Fig. 11.2 Mammograms A, mediolateral and B, craniocaudal showing a well-defined low-density mass in the lower central breast. The appearance is of a benign lesion, such as a cyst or fibroadenoma. Such an appearance has a low chance of being caused by a malignancy.

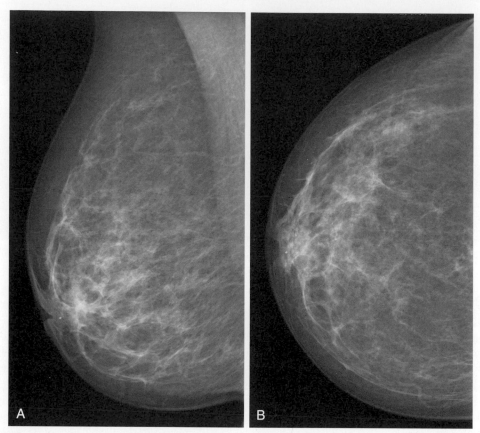

Fig. 11.3 Mammograms (A, mediolateral and B, craniocaudal) showing an ill-defined low density mass in the retroareolar region. Although it is possible this is caused by a cyst, a papilloma, or an abscess, a carcinoma cannot be excluded. Ultrasound confirmed the presence of an abscess.

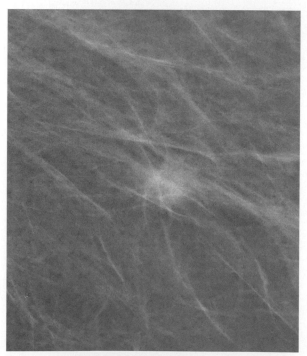

Fig. 11.4 Localized mammographic image showing an ill-defined mass. Although it is possible this is caused by a cyst, a papilloma, or a fibroadenoma, a carcinoma cannot be excluded. Ultrasound confirmed the presence of a breast cancer.

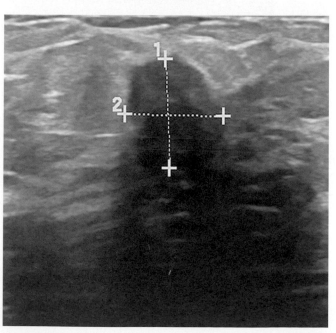

Fig. 11.5 Ultrasound image showing a malignant mass. The mass has an irregular outline with posterior shadowing is taller (line 1) than it is wide (line 2).

A spiculate mass (Fig. 11.6) is defined as an irregular mass with ill-defined margins and surrounding parenchymal reaction, producing spicules and tentacles (representing a combination of pulling in of surrounding fibrous bands and outgrowths of the cancer into the surrounding breast). Spiculate lesions should always be considered malignant until proven otherwise.

Architectural Distortion

Architectural distortion (Fig. 11.7) is defined as distortion of the normal breast parenchymal pattern. It is commonly seen

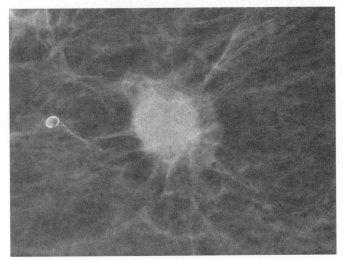

Fig. 11.6 Localized mammographic image showing a spiculate mass. Such an appearance has a high chance of being caused by invasive carcinoma. Ultrasound confirmed a carcinoma.

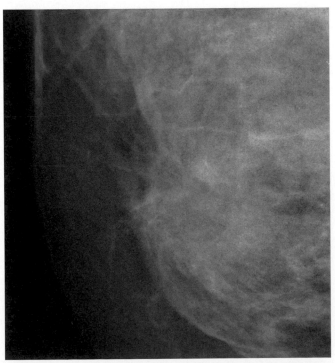

Fig. 11.7 Localized mammogram demonstrating an architectural distortion. The normal parenchyma of the breast is being "drawn" into a central focus.

in association with an ill-defined mass lesion, an appearance strongly suspicious of an invasive breast carcinoma. Architectural distortion may also occur on its own when its cause may be equally sinister.

On mammography, apparent deformity is often produced by the summation of normal overlapping shadows.

The differential diagnosis of architectural distortion without an associated mass lies between a radial scar (complex sclerosing lesion) and carcinoma. The presence or absence of associated microcalcification does not alter this differential.

Asymmetry

Asymmetry is a nonspecific sign (Fig. 11.8). Asymmetry is common and is rarely the sole sign of malignancy. The large majority of asymmetrical densities simply represent normal breast tissue (asymmetrical involution). Asymmetry is defined as "a focal area of increased density," often interspersed with varying amounts of fatty tissue and often demonstrating concave margins. In the absence of any clinical finding, asymmetry without any other associated mammographic features is very unlikely to be of significance but can occasionally be associated with lobular breast cancer; therefore further imaging investigation is not unreasonable.

Microcalcifications

The majority of microcalcifications in the breast are associated with benign breast conditions (e.g., sclerosing adenosis, fibrocystic change, duct ectasia). To select the microcalcifications that represent malignant disease is not an easy task. A careful analysis of the mammographic appearances may allow microcalcifications to be divided into benign and high-risk of malignancy groups. These features include morphology, density, distribution, and change with magnification and change with time (Table 11.2).

Round and ring calcifications are usually benign. Granular and casting microcalcifications in a ductal distribution are much more suspicious. Clusters of calcifications are more likely to signify malignancy, whereas widespread, scattered particles are more likely to be associated with benign changes. The number of calcifications within a cluster is of no value in differential diagnosis, but the shape of a cluster can be of help. A spherical or oval cluster is likely to be benign, but any other shape is suggestive of malignancy. The only occasion when numbers of calcifications may assist in the differentiation of benign from malignant disease is following magnification. Should magnification reveal an increase in the number of calcific particles within the area of previously seen calcifications, then the chance of malignancy is increased. If extra calcifications are visualized outside the area, then the chances of malignancy are lessened. Should there be no increase in the number of particles visible, then benign disease is likely to be the cause.

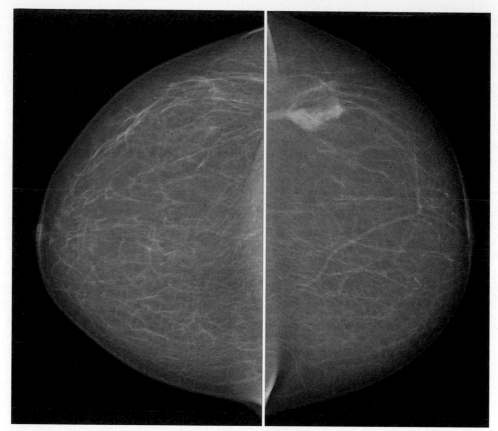

Fig. 11.8 Craniocaudal projections showing asymmetry between the breasts. Such an appearance without additional mammographic features has a low chance of representing malignancy and is almost always a benign/normal finding. Ultrasound confirmed an "island" of normal glandular tissue.

TABLE 11.2 **Features Helpful in Defining the Nature of Microcalcifications**		
Feature	**Benign**	**Malignant**
Cluster shape	Round	Irregular
Particle size	Large	Small
Particle shape	Round	Irregular (rods and branches)
Particle density	Low	Dense or mixed
Number after magnification	Same or widely distributed	More in cluster

BENIGN BREAST CONDITIONS

Benign Breast Changes

Hormonal changes have an effect in the breast leading to a large variety of findings histologically and radiologically. This ranges from initial breast development through normal cyclical activity associated with most of the premenopausal years through to involutionary change as a woman approaches the menopause. These variations are normal, often bilateral and symmetrical, and usually symptomless. In the past, numerous names have been used to describe the various entities within this group of conditions—chronic mastitis, cystic mastitis, mastopathy, and fibroadenosis being among the more common. In the absence of evidence of any disease process, some considered it better to discard the term disease completely. Because this whole group of conditions can be simply explained on the basis of variations (aberrations) of normal processes, it is now common practice to call them collectively "benign breast changes."

Classification of Benign Breast Lesions

Mammographic appearances vary according to the structures which are mainly affected. The two most commonly involved are the larger ducts and terminal ductolobular units (TDLUs).

Benign epithelial breast lesions can be classified histologically into three categories: nonproliferative, proliferative without atypia, and atypical hyperplasia. The categorization is based upon the degree of cellular proliferation (rapid increase in number of normal looking cells) and atypia (abnormal but not cancerous).

Nonproliferative Breast Lesions

Nonproliferative epithelial lesions are generally not associated with an increased risk of breast cancer. As noted already, terms such as duct ectasia, fibrocystic changes, chronic cystic mastitis, and mammary dysplasia refer to nonproliferative lesions and are not useful clinically, as they encompass a heterogeneous group of diagnoses. The most common nonproliferative breast lesions are breast cysts.

Other nonproliferative lesions include hamartomas, lipomas, papillary apocrine change, epithelial-related calcifications, and mild hyperplasia of the usual type. Apocrine metaplasia (also referred to as a "benign epithelial alteration") is also a nonproliferative change that is secondary to some form of irritation, typically associated with a breast cyst.

Mammographic Appearances Associated With Common Nonproliferative Breast Lesions

Cysts

Cystic changes in the breast are very common. During normal cyclical activity, the cells lining the TDLUs increase in size and an increase in the diameter of the lobules is often seen associated with this. On occasions, this dilatation is to such a degree that cysts are formed. Any condition, in which the rate of secretion by the epithelial cells exceeds the capacity of the duct to drain the lobule, will cause the lobule to dilate and a cyst will form. Some cysts may dilate to a size which renders them visible on imaging either as a well-defined mass on mammography or as an anechoic lesion on US (Fig. 11.9). A few of them may dilate further and become palpable. Should one or two cysts be palpable within a breast then it is highly likely that more will be demonstrated by mammography or US.

An inflammatory reaction may also occur around dilated TDLUs and lead to fibrosis. The combination of fibrosis and cyst formation is known as fibrocystic change. This may be visualized on a mammogram as an increase in density, or on US examination as a diffuse increase in small echoes in the affected region, together with cysts of various sizes.

Cyst contents often have a high concentration of calcium which may precipitate to form minute dust-like particles

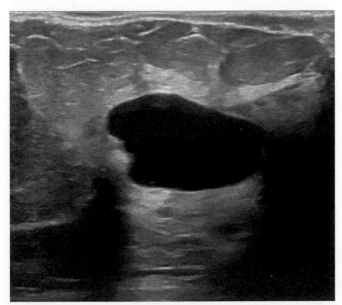

Fig. 11.9 Ultrasound image showing a anechoic "oval" structure with distal brightness and edge attenuation. The appearances are those of a simple cyst.

suspended in the cyst fluid. This is known as milk of calcium. The calcium particles sink to the bottom of the cyst and, when viewed on a craniocaudal (CC) projection, are seen as a soft density with a rounded margin. When viewed on a medial-lateral or lateral medial projection, the density will be crescentic, having a straight upper margin. This appearance is known as the "tea cup" sign, and is characteristic and diagnostic of fibrocystic change.

Duct Ectasia

Occasionally, dilated ducts can become filled with debris which may calcify, a feature that is often visible on a mammogram (broken needle appearance). Duct contents may escape into the surrounding tissue, exciting an inflammatory reaction (periductal mastitis). On occasions, the end result of this process can be visualized on a mammogram as small, calcified plates surrounding and running alongside the ducts, giving a characteristic "pipe stem" appearance (Fig. 11.10). Calcifications are the most common mammographic manifestation of duct ectasia.

Fibroadenoma

Proliferation of both the epithelial and stromal elements of the TDLU can give rise to a localized well-defined mass known as a fibroadenoma. These masses are often too small to give symptoms and may be detected as incidental findings on mammography performed for other reasons. Fibroadenomas that grow large enough to produce a palpable lump most commonly occur in women in their 20s and 30s. They are well defined, ovoid lesions of rubbery consistency. New fibroadenomas do not appear, nor are existing ones seen to grow in size, in postmenopausal women, except in women who are having HRT.

On mammography, a fibroadenoma is seen as a mass which displaces the normal tissue, has smooth, rounded, well-defined margin, but no specific characteristic features (Fig. 11.11). Calcification commonly occurs in fibroadenomata, particularly in those which have been present for some time. When calcification does occur, then it often has an absolutely characteristic "popcorn" appearance on mammography (Fig. 11.12).

Coarse "popcorn" calcification is often associated with a longstanding fibroadenoma. Fibroadenoma can be difficult to distinguish from cysts on mammography; US is important in these cases. Fibroadenoma usually shows a well-defined, oval, homogeneous, hypoechoic mass with either no distal effect or distal bright up (Fig. 11.13).

Proliferative Breast Lesions

When the cells in the ducts or lobules are growing faster than normal, but the cells look normal, one of a number of proliferative breast lesions without atypia occurs. Having one of these conditions may slightly increase the risk of breast cancer. Examples include ductal hyperplasia, lobular hyperplasia, papillomas, complex fibroadenomas, sclerosing adenosis, and radial scar. Proliferative lesions with atypia occur when cells in the ducts or lobules are growing faster than normal and

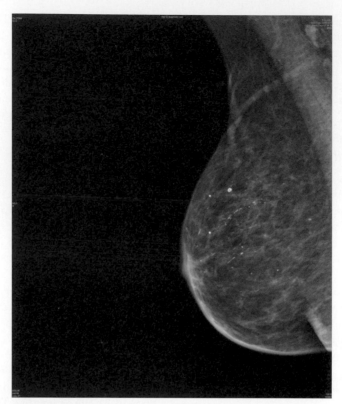

Fig. 11.10 The "pipe stem" appearance of calcification associated with duct ectasia.

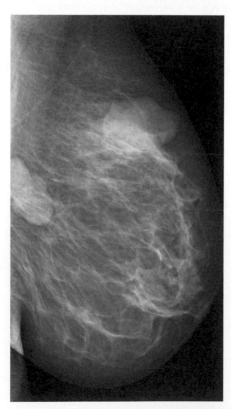

Fig. 11.11 Mammographic image showing well-defined masses. Biopsy confirmed fibroadenoma.

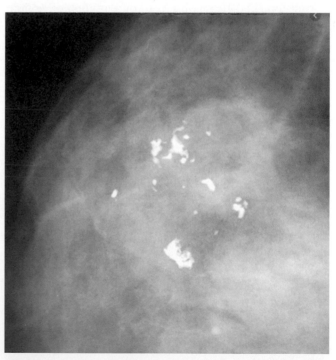

Fig. 11.12 Coarse "popcorn" calcification often associated with a longstanding fibroadenoma.

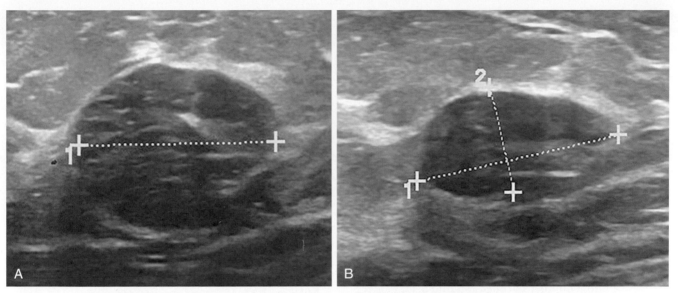

Fig. 11.13 Ultrasound images (A and B) of fibroadenomas. An oval shaped homogenous mass that is wider (line 1) than it is tall (line 2). Core biopsy is usually indicated to confirm a fibroadenoma.

look abnormal. The specific conditions are atypical ductal hyperplasia and atypical lobular hyperplasia.

Proliferative lesions, particularly those with atypia, carry a greater breast cancer risk; this varies according to the histologic appearance, age at diagnosis, and family history. These lesions are considered risk markers, rather than being premalignant, because any cancers which may subsequently develop are not necessarily in the area of atypia and may occur in the contralateral (other) breast. They are usually removed by either image-guided vacuum excision or surgical excision depending on the lesion type. The breast screening program provides guidance in their assessment guidelines.

Mammographic Appearances Associated With Common Proliferative Breast Lesions

Sclerosing Lesions

The central part of the lesion shows fibrosis which contracts to form a scar which causes distortion of the normal surrounding architecture (radial scar). Calcifications are a commonly associated feature as is the absence of a focal mass at the center of the distortion. Typically, the lesions are discoid in shape, and are therefore more easily visible "en face" than if projected end on. This may result in a radial scar being more clearly visible in one projection than another (Fig. 11.14). Screening mammography will detect about two radial scars in every 1000 women screened. If a large area is involved in this sclerosing, deforming process then the condition is called a complex sclerosing lesion. The mass of tissue so formed may feel hard and fixed to the surrounding tissues on palpation and can therefore be mistaken for a carcinoma.

Papillary Lesions

Papillary lesions which arise within breast ducts often appear as well-defined opacities on mammography, whereas mammographic features of sclerosing adenosis/radial scars are

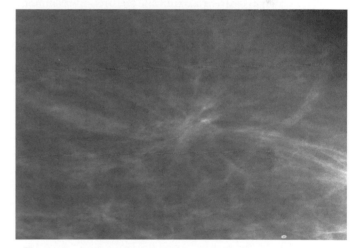

Fig. 11.14 A subtle distortion often associated with a radial scar.

varied and include ill-defined masses, architectural distortion, and suspicious microcalcification. Appearances can be indistinguishable from that caused by a carcinoma.

Even if these lesions are proven to be benign, they have uncertain malignant potential which may indicate further management.

MALIGNANT AND POTENTIALLY MALIGNANT CONDITIONS

What Is Breast Cancer?

Cancer and carcinoma are terms used to describe uncontrolled overgrowth of abnormal cells, a disease process which may ultimately threaten the life of the host. Breast carcinoma is a term used collectively to describe a heterogeneous group of malignant conditions, the vast majority of which arise in the epithelial cells in the terminal duct lobular unit. Breast cancer can be divided into two main types: in situ carcinoma, which is contained within the ducts or lobules, and invasive carcinoma, which has spread out of the ducts or lobules through the basement membrane into the adjacent breast tissue. Invasive carcinoma has the potential to spread via the bloodstream or lymphatic vessels to other parts of the body (metastatic breast carcinoma). In situ carcinoma is divided into low, intermediate, and high grade. As it often presents as asymptomatic microcalcification on mammography, it became more prevalent since the advent of breast screening. Historically, all in situ disease was thought to be precancerous, with the potential to develop into invasive disease and shorten life. Treatment was either wide local excision or mastectomy. More recent research suggests that low and even intermediate ductal carcinoma in situ (DCIS) will not be problematic within the woman's lifetime and current research is assessing the safety in not removing some types of DCIS.

There are also a number of other conditions that are recognized to be precancerous (Table 11.3). They range from those with very little risk of progression to malignancy to those with a highly significant risk. These conditions, except for DCIS, have no clearly recognizable features on mammography to distinguish them from the benign processes already described. Mammography has a very limited role in the assessment and management of these potentially malignant conditions.

Types of Breast Cancer

A simple classification of both in situ and invasive breast cancer is shown in Table 11.4. Lobular carcinoma in situ (LCIS) has no identifiable features on mammography and is almost always an incidental finding in a biopsy carried out for another reason. LCIS is a risk factor for breast cancer in either breast. By contrast, DCIS frequently shows characteristic mammographic features, the most common of which is microcalcification. Invasive cancers usually arise directly from an area of DCIS.

The proportion of the different types of breast cancer detected at screening differs from that seen in women of the same age with symptomatic breast cancer. Subtypes which carry a better prognosis, sometimes referred to as special types, are more likely to be found by screening. This is for two

TABLE 11.4 Pathologic Classification of Carcinoma of the Breast

Main Classification	Subclassification
Ductal	In situ (DCIS)
	Invasive
Lobular	In situ (LCIS)
	Invasive
Medullary	
Special types	Tubular
	Papillary
	Mucinous
	Invasive cribriform
Mixed	
Rare Types	Spindle cell
	Metaplastic
	Apocrine
	Secretory
	Inflammatory

DCIS, Ductal carcinoma in situ; *LCIS*, lobular carcinoma in situ.

reasons: first, screening mammography detects breast cancer at an earlier stage, before it is palpable; and second, special-type tumors often produce features that are easier to detect on mammography.

Invasive Cancer Grade

The grading of invasive breast cancer is determined by the number of tubules, the number of mitoses, and the degree of nuclear pleomorphism demonstrated histologically. Tumors with a low degree of nuclear pleomorphism and low counts of mitoses and high counts of tubule formation are low-grade tumors. Tumors with no tubule formation, high in mitotic counts, and a high degree of pleomorphism are high grade. The histologic grade of an invasive cancer is the major intrinsic prognostic factor. High-grade tumors carry a poor prognosis where low-grade tumors carry a good prognosis. Cancers detected by mammographic screening are on average of a lower histologic grade than cancers presenting symptomatically. Mammographically high-grade invasive cancers present as either an ill-defined or spiculate mass which is commonly associated with casting-type calcification. Low-grade invasive cancers normally present as a small spiculate mass or architectural distortion and calcification is much less common.

The Mammographic Features of Breast Cancer According to Pathologic Types
Ductal Carcinoma In Situ

DCIS accounts for around 20% of screen-detected cancers compared with 5% of symptomatic cancers. This is because DCIS rarely gives rise to clinical symptoms, whereas its primary mammographic sign, microcalcification, is easy to detect at a preclinical stage. DCIS may be broadly divided into high-grade, intermediate-grade, and low-grade, all most commonly seen as microcalcifications.

TABLE 11.3 Histologic Terms Used to Describe the Transition From Normal Epithelium to Malignancy

Histologic Term	Increasing Risk of Developing Invasive Carcinoma
Normal epithelial hyperplasia (ductal and lobular)	
Atypical lobular hyperplasia	
Atypical ductal hyperplasia	
Lobular carcinoma in situ	
Ductal carcinoma in situ	

The microcalcifications typical of high-grade DCIS (casts, branching, and granular microcalcifications in a ductal distribution) are produced by calcification of necrotic tissue in the center of the affected ducts (Fig. 11.15). The extent of mammographic microcalcification in high-grade DCIS correlates well with the actual extent of the disease. High-grade DCIS is an aggressive process with 30% to 50% of cases progressing to invasive carcinoma within 5 years. Paget disease of the nipple, which usually presents as nipple inflammation similar to eczema, is a form of DCIS.

The microcalcifications associated with low-grade DCIS tend to be better defined and form as pearl-like laminated structures within the mucin-containing intercellular spaces. These calcifications may be morphologically indistinguishable from those associated with benign breast change. They are therefore more difficult to recognize as malignant, their distribution being the most important feature. Malignant microcalcifications tend to be arranged in linear, irregular, or V-shaped clusters, whereas benign microcalcifications tend to be arranged in rounded clusters. Low-grade DCIS has a risk of invasion of 40% at 30 years follow-up.

DCIS is also an important feature to document in association with invasive carcinoma as its presence often means breast conservation surgery is not appropriate. Breast-conserving treatment for DCIS requires careful preoperative evaluation, in which mammography plays a very important role. Knowledge of the mammographic spectrum of DCIS is essential for this process.

Invasive Ductal Carcinoma

Invasive ductal carcinoma is the most common histologic type of breast cancer and is often referred to as ductal carcinoma of no specific type. It has a wide spectrum of appearances on mammography, but the most common is spiculate mass (Fig. 11.16). Other less common mammographic features are ill-defined irregular mass, parenchymal distortion, asymmetry, and calcification. The parenchymal distortion is caused by the fibrous reaction causing pulling in of adjacent structures.

Approximately one-third of invasive ductal carcinomas are associated with microcalcification. The combination of a spiculate mass and microcalcification is very strong evidence of malignancy.

Lobular Carcinoma In Situ

LCIS has no specific mammographic features. It is not a true malignancy and should be regarded simply as a risk factor. LCIS itself rarely calcifies but is often associated with benign processes which produce microcalcification. LCIS is usually an incidental finding in biopsy specimens.

Invasive Lobular Carcinoma

Invasive lobular carcinoma cannot be distinguished from ductal carcinoma by its mammographic appearances. The majority of lobular carcinomas show very similar features to ductal carcinoma, with a spiculate mass being the most common appearance although often more subtle (Fig. 11.17). A few produce little or no mammographic abnormality despite being large in size; therefore MRI is often required

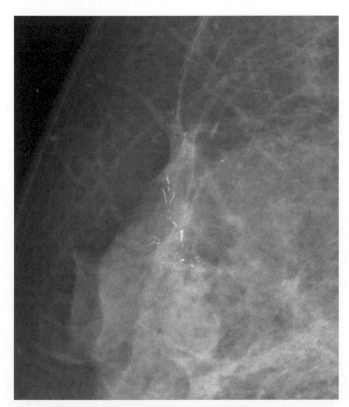

Fig. 11.15 Irregular shaped cluster of microcalcifications. The calcifications themselves show marked pleomorphism and a ductal distribution. The appearances are those of high-grade ductal carcinoma in situ.

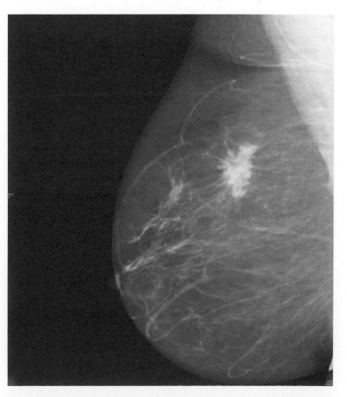

Fig. 11.16 Invasive ductal carcinoma presenting as a spiculate mass.

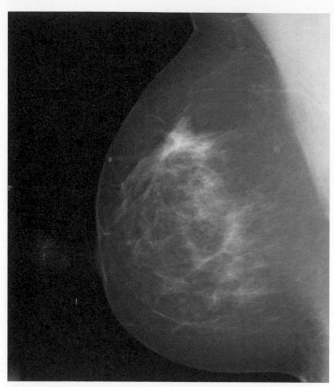

Fig. 11.17 The more subtle mammographic appearances associated with an invasive lobular carcinoma.

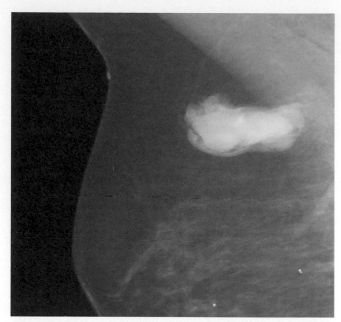

Fig. 11.18 A mucinous carcinoma. Partially well-defined but more dense than a benign mass.

to establish extent of disease. Microcalcifications is less commonly seen in association with lobular carcinoma.

Medullary Carcinoma

Medullary carcinoma is rare. It is most often demonstrated as a partly well defined, dense mass lesion without architectural distortion (Fig. 11.18). As such, it may mimic a benign lesion, such as a cyst or fibroadenoma.

Mucinous Carcinoma

Mucinous carcinoma is another uncommon tumor which also produces a mostly well-defined mass on mammography. Its mucinous content can result in distal enhancement on US, a feature usually associated with benign lesions.

Tubular Carcinoma

Tubular carcinoma is found much more commonly as a result of screening. Tubular carcinoma typically produces architectural distortion which is more extensive than would be expected for the size of the central tumor mass. This feature is easy to detect on mammography and, as a result, many can be detected at a small size. Tubular carcinomas often have features that are indistinguishable on mammography from radial scar or complex sclerosing lesions. Some carcinomas have features of more than one tumor type. The most common of such lesions are tubular mixed cancers with features and prognosis between these of tubular cancer and ductal carcinomas of no specific type.

SUMMARY

The following are some general observations about mammographic interpretation.

- Well-defined masses are very likely to be benign.
- Ill-defined masses deserve careful assessment.
- Spiculate masses and focal areas of architectural distortion should be regarded as malignant until proven otherwise.
- Asymmetries are rarely important.
- Microcalcifications are often difficult to evaluate and may represent DCIS with or without an invasive focus.
- A spiculate mass with pleomorphic microcalcification is highly suspicious of malignancy.

The secret of success in the diagnosis of breast problems is careful clinical and imaging assessment with judicious use of core biopsy. Assessment should not stop until a definitive outcome is obtained.

FURTHER READING

Andolina, V., aLille, S. (2011). *Mammographic imaging: a practical guide* (3rd ed.). Philadelphia: Wolters Kluwer/Lippincott Williams & Wilkins Health.

Barkhausen, J., Rody, A., Schafer. F.K.W. (2016). *Digital breast tomosynthesis: technique and cases.* New York: Thieme.

Bland, K.I., Copeland, E.M., Klimberg, V.S., Gradishar, W.J. (2017). The breast: comprehensive management of benign and malignant diseases. In *The Breast: Comprehensive Management of Benign and Malignant Diseases.* Elsevier Inc.

Borrelli, C., Cohen, S., Duncan, A., et al. (2016). NHSBSP; Clinical guidance for breast cancer screening assessment, publication 49. Public Health England. Available at: https://associationofbreastsurgery.org.uk/media/1414/nhs-bsp-clinical-guidance-for-breast-cancer-screening-assessment.pdf (Accessed 20/04/20).

Chinyama, C.N. (2014) *Benign breast diseases: radiology - pathology - risk assessment.* Springer Science and Business Media.

Covington, M.F., Pizzitola, V.J., Lorans, R., et al. (2018). The future of contrast-enhanced mammography. *AJR. American Journal of Roentgenology*, 210(2), 292.

Dixon, J.M. (2012). *ABC of breast diseases.* Blackwell Pub.

D'Orsi CJ, Sickles EA, Mendelson EB, Morris EA, et al. (2013). *ACR BI-RADS® Atlas, breast imaging reporting and data system.* Reston, VA: American College of Radiology.

Feldman, E.D., Oppong, B.A., Willey, S.C. (2012). Breast cancer screening: Clinical, radiologic, and biochemical. *Clinical Obstetrics and Gynaecology, 55*(3). Available at: https://doi.org/10.1097/GRF.0b013e31825ca884 (Accessed 17/04/20).

Giess, C.S., Frost, E.P., Birdwell, R.L. (2012). Difficulties and errors in diagnosis of breast neoplasms. *Seminars in Ultrasound, CT and MRI*, 33(4).

Gilbert, F.J., Tucker, L., Young, K.C. (2016). Digital breast tomosynthesis (DBT): a review of the evidence for use as a screening tool. *Clinical Radiology*, 71(2), 141–150).

Gunderman, R.B., McNeive, L.R. (2014). Is structured reporting the answer? *Radiology*, 273(1), 7–9.

Haneuse, S., Buist, D.S.M., Miglioretti, D.L., et al. (2011). Mammographic interpretive volume and diagnostic mammogram interpretation performance in community practice 1. *Radiology*, 262.

Harvey, J., March, D.E (2013) *Making the diagnosis: a practical guide to breast imaging.* Philidelphia: Saunders Elsevier.

Hogg, P., Kelly, J., Mercer, C. eds (2015). *Digital mammography. A holistic approach.* Switzerland: Springer International Publishing.

Johnson, K., Sarma, D., Hwang, E.S. (2015). Lobular breast cancer series: Imaging. *Breast Cancer Research*, 17(1).

Kim, G., Phillips, J., Cole, E., et al. (2019). Comparison of contrast-enhanced mammography with conventional digital mammography in breast cancer screening: a pilot study. (Report). *Journal of the American College of Radiology*, 16(10), 1456.

Kopans, D.B. (2006). *Breast Imaging* (3rd ed). Baltimore, Maryland: Lippincott Williams & Wilkins.

Maxwell, A.J., Ridley, N.T., Rubin, G., Wallis, M.G., Gilbert, F.J., Michell, M.J. (2009). The Royal College of Radiologists Breast Group breast imaging classification. *Clinical Radiology*, 64(6), 624–627.

Nass, S.J., Patlak, M. (2015). Assessing and improving the interpretation of breast images. In Nass, S.J., Patlak, M. eds. *Assessing and improving the interpretation of breast images* (1st ed.). National Academies Press.

Nori, J, Kaur, M. (2018). *Contrast-enhanced digital mammography (CEDM).* Springer International.

The Royal College of Radiologists. (2019). *Guidance on screening and symptomatic breast imaging 4th edition.* November. Clinical Radiology. Available at: https://www.rcr.ac.uk/system/files/publication/field_publication_files/bfcr199-guidance-on-screening-and-symptomatic-breast-imaging.pdf (Accessed 20/04/20).

Shetty, M.K. ed. (2014). *Breast cancer screening and diagnosis: a synopsis.* New York: Springer.

Shiffman, M. (2009). Breast augmentation. In Shiffman M.A. ed. *Breast augmentation* (1st ed.), pp. 1–672). Springer Berlin Heidelberg.

Sinn, H.P., Kreipe, H. (2013). A brief overview of the WHO classification of breast tumors. *Breast Care*, 8(2), 149–154.

Tabár, L., Tot, T., Dean, P.B. (2008). *Crushed stone-like calcifications: the most frequent malignant type: Vol. Breast can.* Thieme.

Tagliafico, A., Houssami, N., Calabrese, M. eds. (2016). *Digital breast tomosynthesis: a practical approach.* Switzerland: Springer.

Breast Screening

OBJECTIVES

This chapter outlines:
- The principles behind population screening
- How breast screening fits into this and how the program has evolved
- Why mammography is the imaging choice for breast screening
- New digital techniques
- Triple assessment in screening
- Monitoring the quality of the service

PRINCIPLES OF SCREENING

Screening identifies apparently healthy people who may be at increased risk of a disease or condition, enabling earlier diagnosis and treatment and therefore potentially improved outcomes. National population screening programs are implemented in the National Health Service (NHS) on the advice and recommendations of the UK National Screening Committee (UK NSC). They are funded by NHS England via a protected budget agreed by the Department of Health and Social Care. They target large population groups to assess for early signs of cancer or disease.

The large majority of people who attend population screening will be found to have no abnormality. No screening test is 100% effective. It is important to recognize that some people will be screened who have the condition and it will not be detected. Similarly, others may receive a "false positive result" and find themselves subjected to further tests or possibly more invasive procedures that prove to be unnecessary. Screening programs are effectively judged on whether the benefits to those who are treated earlier outweigh the harms to those who are treated unnecessarily, or who are subject to unnecessary anxiety. The ultimate aim of a screening program is to reduce mortality from the disease.

Before screening for any disease becomes clinical practice, it is important that a number of questions be addressed to confirm that screening will be effective. The main points are set out subsequently:
- The condition/disease should be an important health problem in terms of frequency and/or severity.
- The screening test should be simple, safe, precise, and should be acceptable to the target population.
- There should be an agreed policy on the further diagnostic investigation of individuals with a positive test result and on the choices available to those individuals.
- There should be evidence that diagnosis and treatment before the disease is symptomatic leads to better outcomes for the screened individual compared with usual care.
- There should be evidence from high-quality randomized controlled trials that the screening program is effective in reducing mortality or morbidity.
- The benefit gained by individuals from the screening program should outweigh any harms, for example from overdiagnosis, overtreatment, false positives, false reassurance, uncertain findings, and complications.
- The opportunity cost of the screening program (including testing, diagnosis and treatment, administration, training, and quality assurance) should be economically balanced in relation to expenditure on medical care as a whole (value for money).

- There should be a plan for managing and monitoring the screening program and an agreed set of quality assurance standards.
- Adequate staffing and facilities for testing, diagnosis, treatment, and program management should be available before the commencement of the screening program.
- Evidence-based information, explaining the purpose and potential consequences of screening, should be made available to potential participants to assist them in making an informed choice.

The principles discussed all relate to breast screening which began with the aim of a 20% reduction in mortality from breast cancer. Although the program has evolved significantly over the years, the principles and aim are still valid today.

INCIDENCE OF BREAST CANCER

Breast cancer is the most common cancer in women globally. It is the most common cancer in the United Kingdom, affecting more women than men. A woman born after 1960, and living in the United Kingdom, has an estimated 1 in 7 lifetime risk of developing breast cancer, whereas a British man's lifetime risk of developing breast cancer is around 1 in 870. The disease accounts for 15% of all female cancer deaths. A total of 15,000 women die of breast cancer every year in England and Wales. These facts confirm that breast cancer is an important health problem and it has been shown that inviting women aged 50 to 70 years every 3 years prevents around 1300 breast cancer deaths a year.

SCREENING WITH MAMMOGRAPHY

Mammography has been the screening modality used for every randomized-controlled trial that has shown a significant population breast cancer mortality reduction. It is still accepted as the modality of choice for population screening for breast cancer. In the United Kingdom, it is offered to women aged 50 to 70 years, with women over 70 years able to self-refer. It is quick to perform and relatively quick to interpret, however great skill is needed by the mammographer to produce mammograms of optimum quality. This can be technically challenging and some women find the procedure uncomfortable. A woman's first screening examination is known as the prevalent screen, and subsequent screenings are known as incident screens. Prevalent women are more likely to be recalled for assessment, this is most commonly caused by not having previous mammograms to compare with.

The sensitivity of screening mammography can be estimated by comparing the numbers of cancers occurring between normal screening examinations (intervals) with the breast cancer incidence in an age-matched nonscreened population. Such calculations show a 76% decrease in symptomatic breast cancer in the first year following a negative screen. This reduces to 41% and 21% in the second and third years after a negative screen.

Radiation Dose

Mammography uses ionizing radiation and so is theoretically capable of inducing breast cancer. The risk of a radiation-induced cancer for a woman attending full field digital mammographic screening (two views) by the National Health Service Breast Screening Programme (NHSBSP) is between one in 49,000 to one in 98,000 per visit. It is estimated that about 400 to 800 cancers are detected by the NHSBSP for every cancer induced and the mortality benefit of screening exceeds the radiation-induced detriment by about 150:1 to 300:1.

Number of Views

The screening program started with only mediolateral oblique (MLO) mammograms being undertaken. Subsequent evidence helped practice evolve, and led to the addition of craniocaudal (CC) views of each breast to all mammographic screening examinations. Research showed that the second view increased the detection of breast cancer by 24% and reduced the recall rate by 15%. It particularly made a difference in the detection of invasive cancer less than 10 mm in size. Such tumors are those most likely to lead to the mortality benefit associated with screening. The cost was obviously higher than with single view mammography, but owing to the improved screening performance, the introduction of two views was found to be cost effective.

Digital Mammography

The progression of screening with x-ray film to full field digital imaging, with its high resolution and reconstructive algorithms, has allowed much more flexibility in the use of mammography. Digital breast tomosynthesis (DBT) uses a series of low-dose mammography images acquired at different angles over the breast. Resultant digital images are reconstructed into a series of high-resolution 1-mm slices (or thicker slabs) so that any plane of breast is in focus with other structures outside that plane appearing blurred.

Advantages of DBT are:
- Increased invasive cancer detection rate and in most studies decreases the false positive recall rate.
- Unexpected multifocal disease can be demonstrated.
- It increases sensitivity in the dense breast.
- It may help to localize lesions which are seen initially on a single projection only.
- It has the potential to reduce biopsy rate of normal/benign densities present on full field digital mammography which subsequently resolve on DBT.

Disadvantages are:
- It currently has no significant effect on calcification (ductal carcinoma in situ [DCIS]) detection although the performance of newer machines in this area is improving.
- The examination and interpretation time are typically longer than for a standard set of images.
- DBT images are larger data file sizes than standard mammographic images, which can present IT challenges and associated cost implications.

These aspects of its use need to be addressed before it could be considered for population screening and research is ongoing. DBT is currently approved for use within the assessment clinic and for the symptomatic population. Departments with DBT should consider the facility for DBT-guided biopsy for those abnormalities only seen on DBT and not on two-dimensional mammography or ultrasound (US).

Contrast-enhanced spectral mammography (CESM) is another technique enabled by digital mammography. It involves an injection of contrast media, given in much the same way as it is for a computed tomography scan just before the digital mammogram is taken. This yields information about the additional blood supply associated with cancer formation, as well as the usual size and shape changes seen on mammography which can indicate malignancy. This can improve cancer detection and the technique is proving useful to replace magnetic resonance imaging (MRI) in some settings, being cheaper, available in the breast unit and more acceptable to most patients. However, it is not suitable as a mass population screening technique and is currently only used in the symptomatic population.

FEATURES OF BREAST SCREENING

Age and Frequency

Breast screening undertaken in women aged 50 to 59 and 60 to 69 years has historically been shown to significantly reduce mortality in these age groups (28% and 31% respectively). Screening has also been shown to be cost-effective in these age groups as firstly, there is a high breast cancer incidence in this age group (at least 2 times that in women aged 40–49 years) and, secondly, the lead time of screening in these age groups is such that the screening interval does not need to be less than 2 years.

The screening interval (the time between screening examinations) should be less than the lead-time provided by screening. (Lead-time is the time between diagnosis by screening and the time the cancer would have presented clinically.) If the screening interval is too long many interval cancers occur leading to a reduction in the effectiveness of screening. Estimates of the lead-time achieved by mammographic screening in women aged 40 to 49, 50 to 59, and 60 to 69 years are 1.7, 3.3, and 3.8 years respectively. An increase in interval cancers is observed in the third year after screening compared with the first and second years after screening.

Risk

The only risk factors for breast cancer which are currently strong enough to define a population screening population are age and being female. Breast cancer becomes steadily more common with increasing age. However, as the screening program ages, we are able to use evolving evidence to hone the process. This is happening in many aspects of service delivery, not least surrounding the individual's risk of breast cancer. We are fast moving away from the one-size-fits-all

approach to screening and research is currently assessing the need to alter age at onset of screening, its frequency, and the test method used.

Women currently affected by a significant family history of breast cancer and/or a genetic predisposition can be assessed against National Institute for Clinical Excellence (NICE) ± NHSBSP guidelines and receive increased frequency (annual) mammography screening ± MRI screening starting at a younger age. Research is underway to determine any benefits from screening women of current screening age at different intervals based on breast density and genetic assessment. As a result, their screening may be more frequent or less frequent than their current 3 yearly invitation.

Another large study is currently investigating any benefits from adding supplementary imaging to conventional full-field digital mammography (FFDM). Women with dense breasts on current screening are being randomized to receive either CESM, automated whole breast US (ABUS), or abbreviated (shorter) MRI imaging.

The UK Age Extension (AgeX) trial is the largest randomized controlled trial for any condition anywhere in the world and will provide definitive answers on the benefits, or otherwise, of providing an additional screening episode below the age of 50 years and above the age of 70 years. If resources can be made available, a very strong case can be made for extending the trial to include one further round of screening (for women aged 74–76 years). At the time of writing, all women over the age of 70 years are eligible for breast screening and encouraged to self-refer.

Mammography Reporting

The process of reporting has evolved with the screening program; in the beginning, images were reported by only one reader, but double reading quickly became standard practice, in the face of evidence that it can detect more cancers. Double reading with arbitration leads to a 32% to 40% increase in detection of small invasive cancers without increasing the recall rate. Double reading with arbitration is superior to independent double reading or double reading with consensus. Since the introduction of FFDM, artificial intelligence (AI) or computer-aided diagnosis (CAD) became a realistic option. It remains to be seen if single reading with CAD is as effective as double reading.

RECALL FOR ASSESSMENT

Multidisciplinary assessment of screen-detected abnormalities is required to confirm benignity or malignancy quickly and efficiently. Recall for assessment causes considerable anxiety so it is important that the recall rate is kept as low as possible without compromising sensitivity. Recall rates in the NHSBSP should be less than 7% in the prevalent round (initial screening) and less than 5% at incident (subsequent) screens. The anxiety caused by recall is usually short term and rarely has long-standing consequences.

The Assessment Process

Assessment should be carried out by a multidisciplinary team including a responsible assessor (RA), a mammographer, breast care nurse, and pathologist. Triple assessment is performed in a similar fashion as already described in Chapter 8. However, it must be remembered that in the screening setting, assessment is driven by a potential imaging abnormality without a visual or palpable clinical problem to assist with targeting the area for investigation. As such, patients normally undergo further imaging initially in the form of DBT or magnification $\pm$ paddle views. The choice depends on the type and location of the abnormality seen on mammography, the availability of equipment, and the preferences of the RA. What is required should be part of a protocol or be discussed with the mammographer before the case is begun. Clinical examination is then performed in those women where further imaging has confirmed the presence of a significant abnormality. This is followed by targeted US examination of the area highlighted on mammography and needle sampling if necessary.

X-ray guided stereotactic biopsy is used more commonly in the assessment setting as it is the sampling method recommended for microcalcification. Because this is not usually associated with a palpable abnormality, it is often seen on screening mammography and only occasionally as an incidental finding on symptomatic mammograms. Specimen x-rays are used to confirm representative sampling of microcalcifications. Occasionally, all the calcification or the whole of the visible abnormality is removed, particularly using the large bore vacuum sampling. For these cases and whenever correlation is required between the area sampled and the original mammographic abnormality, a marker clip can be deployed at the biopsy site to aid future localization.

The estimate of risk of malignancy of a lesion is based on the combination of imaging and clinical findings. Patient management is based on the most suspicious of these findings. Lesions with a low risk of malignancy are returned to normal screening on the basis of a definitively benign biopsy result. Lesions with a high risk of malignancy are sampled before surgical excision with the aim of making a preoperative diagnosis of malignancy so therapeutic surgery can be facilitated. Preoperative diagnosis rates for malignancy of more than 90% for invasive disease and 75% for DCIS disease can be achieved using core biopsy.

Patient management is best decided at a prospective multidisciplinary meeting where the pathologic, imaging, and clinical findings are discussed before the woman's follow-up appointment. Women should either be returned to normal screening or referred to a breast surgeon for surgical removal of the lesion. Short-term recall is associated with psychologic morbidity, making it a less-favored option.

Localization

Over 50% of screen-detected abnormalities requiring removal for therapeutic or diagnostic purposes will be impalpable and will require marker localization. Marker localizations are performed using either a wire, skin marking (for subtly palpable lesions), carbon granules, magnetic seeds, or isotopes. Marker localization is best performed under US guidance, but stereotaxis is required for lesions not visible on US. The localization procedure is discussed in Chapter 8.

QUALITY ASSURANCE

Mass population screening is a huge undertaking, in terms of the number of women eligible, the number of staff involved in delivering the service, and the processes needed for each step of the screening pathway. For breast cancer screening to be effective, a high standard of performance must be achieved by all facets of the service. From its inception, the NHSBSP has had quality assurance (QA) guidelines for all aspects of the service including radiography, equipment, radiology, pathology, and surgery. QA guidelines for radiologists include cancer detection rates, small cancer detection rates, recall rates, benign biopsy rates, and preoperative diagnosis rates. For mammographers, this includes monitoring the number of repeat images taken and women recalled for technical reasons. There are many publications available online to assist services in achieving targets and optimizing their service.

There are also regional QA teams who are available for day-to-day support. All units submit information regularly to the QA teams who periodically perform multidisciplinary visits to audit all aspects of a unit's performance. Areas of poor performance are identified and must be shown to have been corrected at follow-up visits.

Service data on all aspects of breast screening are also submitted centrally once a year which gives information about the program nationally and allows comparison between regions.

FURTHER READING

Andolina, V., Lille, S. (2011). *Mammographic imaging: a practical guide* (3rd ed.). Philadelphia: Wolters Kluwer/Lippincott Williams & Wilkins Health.

Barkhausen, J., Rody, A., Schafer. F.K.W. (2016) *Digital breast tomosynthesis: technique and cases.* New York: Thieme.

Borrelli, C., Cohen, S., Duncan, A., et al. (2016). NHSBSP; Clinical guidance for breast cancer screening assessment, publication 49. Public Health England. Available at: https://associationofbreast-surgery.org.uk/media/1414/nhs-bsp-clinical-guidance-for-breast-cancer-screening-assessment.pdf (Accessed 20/04/20).

Cancer Research UK. (no date) *Breast Cancer Statistics.* Available at: https://www.cancerresearchuk.org/health-professional/cancer-statistics/statistics-by-cancer-type/breast-cancer (Accessed 21/04/20).

Department of Health. (2013). Public health functions to be exercised by NHS England Service specification No.24 Breast Screening Programme. Available at: www.nationalarchives.gov.uk/doc/open-government-licence/ (Accessed 17/04/20).

Gov.uk. (2013). Evidence review criteria: national screening programmes. [ONLINE] Available at: https://www.gov.uk/government/publications/evidence-review-criteria-national-screening-programmes (Accessed 21/04/20).

Hogg, P., Kelly, J., Mercer, C. eds (2015). *Digital mammography. A holistic approach.* Switzerland: Springer International Publishing.

Johnson, K., Sarma, D., Hwang, E.S. (2015). Lobular breast cancer series: imaging. *Breast Cancer Research*, 17(1), 94.

Kopans, D.B. (2006). *Breast Imaging* (3rd ed). Baltimore, Maryland: Lippincott Williams & Wilkins.

Marmot, M.G., Altman, D.G., Cameron, D.A., Dewar, J.A., Thompson, S.G., Wilcox, M., (2013). The Independent UK. Panel on Breast Cancer Screening. The benefits and harms of breast cancer screening: an independent review: a report jointly commissioned by Cancer Research UK and the Department of Health (England) October. *British Journal of Cancer*, 108, 2205–2240.

NICE (2017) Breast Screening. Scenario: Breast Screening. Available at https://cks.nice.org.uk/breast-screening#!scenario (Accessed 09/03/2020).

NICE (2018) Early and locally advanced breast cancer: diagnosis and management NICE guideline [NG101] July. Available at: https://www.nice.org.uk/guidance/ng101 (Accessed 21/04/20).

Nori, J., Kaur, M. (2018). *Contrast-enhanced digital mammography (CEDM)*. Springer International.

Nyström, L., Wall, S., Rutqvist, L.E., et al. (1993). Breast cancer screening with mammography: overview of Swedish randomised trials. *The Lancet*, 341(8851), 973–978.

Perry, N., Puthaar, E., Broeders, M., et al. (2008). European guidelines for quality assurance in breast cancer screening and diagnosis. Fourth Edition – summary document. *Annals of Oncology* 19(4), 614–622.

Philpotts, L.E., Hooley, R.J. (2017). *Breast tomosynthesis*. Philadelphia: Elsevier.

Public Health England. (2016). NHS Breast Screening Programme. *Guidance on who can undertake arbitration*. Available at: https://assets.publishing.service.gov.uk/government/uploads/system/uploads/attachment_data/file/548405/Arbitration_guidance.pdf (Accessed 21/04/20).

Public Health England. (2017). NHS Breast Screening Programme Guidance for breast screening mammographers. 3rd Ed. Available at: https://assets.publishing.service.gov.uk/government/uploads/system/uploads/attachment_data/file/819410/NHS_Breast_Screening_Programme_Guidance_for_mammographers_final.pdf (Accessed 16/04/20).

Public Health England (2017) Programme Specific Operating Model for Quality Assurance of Breast Screening Programmes. Available at: https://assets.publishing.service.gov.uk/government/uploads/system/uploads/attachment_data/file/653748/BREAST_PSOM.pdf (Accessed 08/04/20).

Public Health England (2017). Reporting, classification and monitoring of interval cancers and cancers following previous assessment. Available at: https://assets.publishing.service.gov.uk/government/uploads/system/uploads/attachment_data/file/801400/Guidance_on_Interval_cancers_Final.pdf (Accessed 08/04/20).

Public Health England. (2019) Illustration of the screening process. [ONLINE] Available at: https://www.gov.uk/guidance/nhs-population-screening-explained#illustration-of-the-screening-process (Accessed 21/04/20).

Sauven, P., Bishop, H., Patnick, J., Walton, J., Wheeler, E., Lawrence, G. (2003). The National Health Service Breast Screening Programme and British Association of Surgical Oncology audit of quality assurance in breast screening 1996-2001. *British Journal of Surgery*, 90(1), 82–87.

The Independent UK Panel on Breast Cancer Screening. (2012). The Benefits and Harms of Breast Cancer Screening: An Independent Review: . October 2012. Available at: https://www.cancerresearchuk.org/sites/default/files/breast-screening-review-exec_0.pdf (Accessed 08/04/20).

The Royal College of Radiologists. (2019). *Guidance on screening and symptomatic breast imaging 4th edition*. November. Clinical Radiology. Available at: https://www.rcr.ac.uk/system/files/publication/field_publication_files/bfcr199-guidance-on-screening-and-symptomatic-breast-imaging.pdf (Accessed 20/04/20).

UK National Screening Committee. (2018). Screening in the UK: making effective recommendations. [ONLINE] Available at: https://assets.publishing.service.gov.uk/government/uploads/system/uploads/attachment_data/file/733226/Screening_in_the_UK_making_effective_recommendations_2017_to_2018.pdf (Accessed 21/04/20).

Wilson, J.M.G., Jungner, G., World Health Organization. (1968). Principles and practice of screening for disease. Available at: https://apps.who.int/iris/bitstream/handle/10665/37650/WHO_PHP_34.pdf (Accessed 21/04/20).

Wilson, R., Liston, J. (eds) (2011). *Quality Assurance Guidelines for Breast Cancer Screening Radiology*. 59. Sheffield: NHS Cancer Screening Programmes. Available at: https://assets.publishing.service.gov.uk/government/uploads/system/uploads/attachment_data/file/764452/Quality_assurance_guidelines_for_breast_cancer_screening_radiology_updated_Dec_2018.pdf (Accessed 20/04/20).

Psychologic Issues and Communication

OBJECTIVES

This chapter outlines:

- Factors affecting those undergoing examinations for breast cancer
- How a variety of communication skills can reduce anxiety levels
- How consideration must be made for men with a diagnosis of breast cancer
- How the mammographer must consider other people's anxiety when their loved one is diagnosed with breast cancer

INFLUENCES ON ANXIETY AND BEHAVIOR ASSOCIATED WITH BREAST CANCER

The Referral Route

Women attend the breast unit via a number of different routes. When invited for routine breast screening, they may well attend a community based mobile unit and only visit the main center if recalled for further assessment of a potential mammographic abnormality identified when the screening images are reported. Other mammography screening services provided are for those women at increased risk of developing breast cancer because they have a significant family history of the disease, sometimes including the identification of a predisposing gene or they have received previously received radiation to the torso as treatment for other cancers. Women are also referred to the breast unit by their doctor when presenting with a potentially significant breast symptom or they may have had a diagnosis and treatment for breast cancer and be on posttreatment surveillance. Whatever the reason, those attending the service are likely to have some anxieties.

For many women, particularly if attending for their first mammogram examination, there is likely to be concern about the procedure itself. Fear of pain and feeling trapped in the machine is not uncommon and some women will feel anxiety and possibly embarrassment about undressing and being handled for positioning. There can also be concern about radiation dose. Even if the examination itself is of minimal concern, all women attending face the possibility of a cancer diagnosis.

Many women who attend for diagnostic procedures will have a benign outcome; however, all will experience similar fears and anxieties until the final outcome is known. Fear and anxiety are natural processes which prepare us for fight or flight. When confronted with a potential threat this primeval drive comes into play. The anxieties relating to a possible breast cancer diagnosis, once triggered, will remain with the individual for some time after the all clear, and in screening, this is viewed as a negative effect of the screening process. For the health care professional dealing with the woman, there will be some sense of the likely significance of a clinical sign or mammographic abnormality. However, for the woman these factors have no significance and each is fearful for themselves and their families. It is important that all health care professionals are aware of this and are alert and sensitive to individual needs.

The anxiety experienced, and how it is manifested, will potentially depend on the type of appointment the woman has. For women attending for routine screening mammography, they are well and arrive by invitation. Whereas the examination and outcome may be of concern, practical aspects of the appointment, such as accessibility of the mobile unit, parking, and wait times may be the elements which cause frustration and anxiety. Women referred with symptoms may be more tolerant of the practicalities of a busy one-stop clinic with fear of a cancer diagnosis the overriding concern. Whatever the main source of anxiety, individuals' reactions and coping styles will vary. Some women will appear nervous, quiet, even sullen, others overly talkative and sometimes even a little aggressive. All can be manifestations of anxiety and staff need to be sensitive to this and react accordingly.

Women who have previously been given a cancer diagnosis and had treatment for the disease will generally be placed on regular follow-up for several years after diagnosis. Their fears will differ to some degree from those in the prediagnostic phase. They will already have faced a cancer diagnosis and considered their own mortality. They will have drawn on their defenses and dealt with the immediate issues. However, these women have to live with cancer for the rest of their lives and this may have long-term effects on their psychologic wellbeing and their quality of life. The majority of women who have previously been diagnosed and treated for breast cancer will have been offered the support of a counseling nurse and/or therapy counselor at diagnosis and through the treatment phase. Women may decline this psychologic support in the early stages but may require it at a later stage. Health care professionals involved in a woman's follow-up should be alert to signs that psychologic support may be needed and report their concerns to the appropriate members of the team.

Outside Influence—Media and Experiential

A woman receiving an invitation to screening, or considering visiting a general practitioner to seek referral for a breast symptom, will already have been subject to a plethora of information relating to breast cancer. She may have had first-hand experience when a family member or close friend has suffered from breast cancer or she may have second-hand experience via relayed stories from friends. She will also have inevitably been subject to vast amounts of information in newspapers, magazines, television, radio, films, the internet, and social media. Some of this information will be accurate and some inaccurate. These experiences and accumulated knowledge will inevitably color the woman's perception of the disease and its likely outcome. It may also affect her attitude on attendance at the breast clinic. Anxiety levels will also be influenced by her own personality together with the phase of her relationship with the breast cancer.

Phases in the Diagnostic Process

Evidence shows that women can experience significant anxiety at every stage of the screening process, including the time between receiving the recall letter and attending the recall appointment. This can be exacerbated if the woman undergoes a biopsy. They may remain concerned about their health for some time after such a procedure. Consequently, a recall to assessment may adversely affect a woman's future attendance at screening appointments.

It is not uncommon for women who have a newly diagnosed cancer to suffer from anxiety and depression, and this may increase over the coming months as the realization of the seriousness of the diagnosis and its implications become apparent. Particularly at risk are those women who have an asymptomatic cancer identified, and to whom the diagnosis is made known over a short time scale. The speed of transference from 'I am normal' to 'I might have a life-threatening disease' is critical. For a woman to have some prior indication of the possible diagnosis before it is actually confirmed seems to be associated with less long-term psychiatric morbidity.

REDUCING ANXIETY

Written Information

Provision of written information prior to an appointment is one way of reducing anxiety. Breast screening programs should take considerable care to provide suitable and accurate information for women invited to attend. This generally provides sufficient information about the risks and benefits of screening and something about the test itself. This places the invitation into a factually accurate context and enables women to make an informed decision. Other breast diagnostic services should also provide some written information relating to the appropriate clinic whether this be symptomatic, family history, or follow-up. Information included might be waiting times, what to wear, where to park, who can come with them, likely tests, and the professional team. All of these can help reduce anxiety about the process and procedures and may go some way toward putting their individual risk into some degree of rational and understandable perspective. Letters can be supplemented by leaflets providing some additional information and perhaps repeating key messages placed in the letter.

Waiting Times

Waiting greatly exacerbates anxiety. Appointment times must be honored and all the waiting periods between different stages of a consultation should be kept to an absolute minimum. A woman should be informed of the reason for, and the likely duration of, any delays. In the case of one-stop clinics where a series of diagnostic tests may be performed, women should be advised of the process together with the potential delays and benefits.

Administrative and Reception Staff

The importance of skillful reception staff should not be underestimated. Women may contact the unit by telephone for a variety of enquiries. In many services, they will also be the first representatives of the team to meet the woman on attendance. It is helpful if reception staff have some knowledge and understanding of the anxieties women may experience and how to deal with them. It is also important that reception staff feel able to alert other staff to potential problems and to call on other staff to deal with specific issues. This will enable reception staff to respond to a woman's needs in a truly effective way and to enable them to recognize women who may need additional support.

Communication of Results

Communication is of paramount importance. A woman should be given a full explanation of what any procedure entails before it is performed and it should be ensured that she understands. At the conclusion she should be told when the results will be available, and how they will be communicated to her. Information regarding the results should be simply and frankly explained by an appropriately trained team member, who should also make her aware of the implications. Again it should be ensured that she understands this explanation.

Women who are finally given a diagnosis of cancer should always be provided with expert emotional support. Common practice is for "bad news" to be given by an appropriately trained team member with a breast care or counseling nurse in attendance. The initial discussion is still regarded as the most significant communication for the woman, but the expert counselor can help clarify several issues and will be trained to identify psychologic cues which may indicate that the woman is not coping well. The NHSBSP advocates a psychological assessment at diagnosis consisting of a 1 to 5 score pre- and post-assessment where 1 is the woman feeling calm and 5 very anxious. This practice is often mirrored in the symptomatic service. In addition, women often undergo a holistic needs assessment at diagnosis, mid, and end of treatment allowing for further psychological intervention if necessary.

MAMMOGRAPHY PRACTITIONERS AND COMMUNICATION

Different types of mammography examinations are likely to raise anxiety levels by differing degrees. The potentially least worrying mammogram for a woman will be one taken as part of routine screening, but even so multiple factors may cause anxiety associated with the examination. This anxiety is reduced soon after the screening episode. Women who are recalled for assessment may then experience higher levels of anxiety but once they have a normal result, most are reassured. A small percentage may have continued high levels of anxiety, which may result in them seeking advice from their general practitioner.

All those individuals who are involved in breast disease diagnosis and management will inevitably have their attitudes influenced by breast cancer. Resulting from the increased importance of mammography in the management of breast cancer, mammographers are now preeminent in this group. Therein lies a benefit and a danger. Being aware of the background, a mammographer can more readily appreciate the woman's attitude to her problems. However, the mammographer should realize that their own perceptions are affected and should not identify too closely with the woman. They should maintain a professional attitude and a degree of authority.

The mammographer is placed in very close physical contact with a woman during the examination; not only is there potential embarrassment and a significant "intrusion into personal space" but the technique required to perform a mammogram can be likened to an embrace. It follows that this degree of intimacy places a particular responsibility upon the mammographers who should be sensitive to the psychologic state of the woman, and be prepared to give whatever support may be necessary. To accomplish this, it is essential to perform the examination in an efficient, confident manner, being as physically gentle as is consistent with the production of a high-quality mammogram, and simultaneously expressing obvious empathy and a caring attitude.

It is also caused by the intimacy of the examination that women may bring issues previously hidden to the fore. These may be issues of a personal nature and in a routine screening examination this can be quite a common occurrence. It provides a chance for the woman to talk to someone fully and frankly about an issue which they will not necessarily share with others. In examinations where anxiety levels relate to breast cancer, the woman may openly express these fears.

Personal Issues

Mammographers are trained to be experts in their area of clinical practice. This puts the mammographer at an advantage over the women. She is likely to perceive the practitioner as more powerful and to undertake the test will generally be compliant with the requests of the mammographer and have respect for their professional expertise. When an issue of a personal nature is brought to the mammographer's attention, it is important to remember that in this area the mammographer is no longer the expert. There is essentially a change in dynamics of the relationship. As a practitioner performing an examination, the mammographer is the expert; in terms of personal lives only the woman can be the expert.

Although, as a general rule, mammographers do not act as professional counselors, on occasions they are called upon to use counseling skills. It is important to remember that counseling skills rely heavily on listening skills and the use of open questions. For the woman, the expression of, and verbalization of, the issue may well be what provides the relief, albeit temporarily, to the problem raised. A benefit of the relationship with the mammographer is that they are independent of their normal life, will respect confidentiality, and will not judge. The mammographer in this situation should not give advice but simply listen, reflect, and clarify.

MEN WITH BREAST SYMPTOMS

As discussed in Chapter 7, breast cancer in men is very rare; however rates have risen over the last 20 years throughout the world. In addition, benign breast conditions, such as gynecomastia, are common; therefore health care professionals must be aware of the potential associated psychologic concerns.

Diagnostic procedures for men with symptoms generally follow the same approach as for women; however there is little research on the psychosocial impact of being diagnosed with a predominantly female disease. Factors, such as shock, poor body image, and traumatic stress symptoms, have been reported, but there are few recommendations on the appropriate management of these.

Evidence suggests that although men experience excellent care, the clinical setting can make them feel marginalized and stigmatized; therefore mammographers must be aware that the male patient may be experiencing similar anxieties as their female counterparts, as well as considering their potential embarrassment regarding having a "woman's" examination.

BREAST CANCER ISSUES

Given the intimacy of mammography and that it is often the first clinical test performed, anxieties about the outcome may be expressed very readily. Information that the woman has not requested should not be offered. However, eliciting whether more information is required is entirely appropriate and leaves the choice to the women. This allows the woman to seek information but only when she is ready to cope with potential answers. To ask "Is there anything you need to know about?" will often precipitate a question which the woman has not completely formulated previously, or is reluctant to ask. In a breast screening follow-up situation, a frequently asked question is "why they have been recalled" This can often be answered by showing the original screening images. This should be left to experienced mammographers who can show the images without being drawn on the potential outcome. The women can then see the difference from one side to the other, realize the importance of having this area assessed, and understand why no answers are immediately available. This knowledge will also help to explain why certain procedures are required and that any associated discomfort is necessary.

It is important that the mammographer is aware of the limitations of their role and is not drawn to answer questions for which there is as yet, no answer. Telling the woman when and how she will get the answers to these questions can be extremely helpful. It cannot be overstressed that great care is necessary before suggesting to a woman that the diagnosis is, or may be, cancer. Communication with the woman on this topic is best left to those who are able to provide the full clinical facts, can discuss the choices available, and have the necessary counseling training to fully support the woman.

This can put enormous pressure on the mammographer. In the meantime, a balance is needed in which neither too much nor too little reassurance is offered.

The mammographer can help women through the various stages of the diagnosis, and treatment when treatment is necessary, by being alert to the individual needs of the women and addressing these to the best of their ability within the context of a multiprofessional team.

THE FAMILY

It has been established for many years that a woman's ability to cope with her anxieties relates strongly to the degree of support she receives. Husbands, partners, and close family members and friends are identified as primary sources of support. Self-help groups, such as voluntary support groups, serve as visible evidence that problems and fears can be overcome. Breast cancer is a family disease. The supportive role of a family has been referred to earlier, but the full effect of a diagnosis of breast cancer on the family may not always be fully appreciated. There is no doubt that healthy family members can be affected by the illness of another family member, with the creation of physical, emotional, and social symptoms. Moreover, the way one family member reacts to an illness can affect the way that another member adjusts. With breast cancer in particular, family members may have considerable difficulty in coping with the emotional ramifications. The occurrence of problems is likely to be greatest during the first year after the development of metastases. Every individual working in a breast diagnostic service has a responsibility to be aware of the problems. The attitude and state of mind of the partner or other family member who accompanies a woman scheduled to have diagnostic tests merits careful consideration. A sympathetic and supportive attitude should be extended to accompanying persons as and when this is judged to be appropriate.

FURTHER READING

Andolina, V., Lille, S. (2011). *Mammographic imaging: a practical guide* (3rd Ed.). Philadelphia: Wolters Kluwer/Lippincott Williams & Wilkins Health.

Barnhart, M.P. (2016). *Breast cancer, an emotional journey: (30 years later)*. Create Space Independent Publishing Platform.

Bontempo, D. (2013). *Breast cancer Mardi Gras: surviving the emotional hurricane and showing my boobs*. AuthorHouse.

Galgut, C. (2010). *The psychological impact of breast cancer: a psychologist's Insights as a patient*. Oxford: Radcliffe publishing Ltd.

Galgut, C. (2013). *Emotional support through breast cancer: the alternative handbook* (1st ed.). London: Radcliffe Publishing limited.

Hogg, P., Kelly, J., Mercer, C. eds (2015). *Digital mammography. A holistic approach.* Switzerland: Springer International Publishing.

Kopans, D.B. (2006). *Breast imaging* (3rd ed). Baltimore, Maryland: Lippincott Williams & Wilkins.

Public Health England. (2017). NHS Breast Screening Programme Guidance for breast screening mammographers. 3rd Ed. Available at: https://assets.publishing.service.gov.uk/government/uploads/system/uploads/attachment_data/file/819410/NHS_Breast_Screening_Programme_Guidance_for_mammographers_final.pdf (Accessed 16/04/20).

Towsley-Cook, D.M., Young, T. A. (2007). *Ethical and legal issues for imaging professionals.* Mosby/Elsevier.

The Multidisciplinary Team

OBJECTIVES

This chapter outlines:
- What a multidisciplinary team is
- A case study to illustrate the function of the multidisciplinary team

INTRODUCTION TO THE MULTIDISCIPLINARY TEAM

All suspected and diagnosed breast cancers are managed by a multidisciplinary approach where each member of the team plays a key role in the diagnosis and management of breast disease.

As one of the first points of contact, the mammographer has a key role in reaching the best outcomes for women and excellent patient experience.

When a woman is investigated for suspected breast cancer or has a diagnosis of breast disease, her case is discussed at a multidisciplinary team (MDT) meeting where an individualized management plan is considered before options are discussed with the woman.

To ensure consistency throughout the diagnostic process most teams will use a designated scoring system to classify the level of suspicion of any abnormality (Table 14.1). The radiology codes do vary between units, for example, "X", "R", or "M" for the mammography. Some units will use "M" or "MR" for magnetic resonance imaging (MRI) scans and "Ax" for ultrasound (US) scans of the axilla, but each department will work to the agreed codes. These grades help guide and direct the most appropriate diagnostic workup and ongoing management of the woman.

The Multidisciplinary Team Meeting

The UK Department of Health defines MDT as "a group of people of different healthcare disciplines which meets together at a given time (whether physically in one place or by video or teleconferencing) to discuss a given patient, and who are each able to contribute independently to the diagnostic and treatment decisions about the patient."

MDTs have been recognized standard practice since the inception of the National Health Service Breast Screening Programme in 1988, and were adopted by all cancer pathways by 1995. The meetings have multiple functions: to ensure that all women receive timely treatment and care from appropriately skilled professionals, that there is continuity of care, and that women get adequate information and support. The teams also facilitate communication between primary, secondary, and tertiary care, as well as collection of reliable data for the benefit of individual women and for audit and research. Teams can monitor adherence to clinical guidelines and can promote the effective use of resources. It can also be an education platform for all participants.

As inferred by the term "multidisciplinary" there is a wide range of health care professionals that participate in these meetings. Each are involved at some stage in the diagnosis and management of breast disease.

Who Attends Multidisciplinary Team Meetings?

Representation will vary depending on each service; however generally there will be a least one of following groups (known as core members):
- *Consultant breast surgeon*
  Breast surgeons oversee the care of people presenting with breast problems, from the initial consultation to the completion of treatment. They advise the team on the surgical management of cases.
- *Consultant radiologist/radiographer*
  The consultant radiologist/radiographer (or responsible assessor as described in Chapter 8) advise the team on the best imaging regime; they direct and coordinate breast imaging tests to ensure all imaging abnormalities are

TABLE 14.1	Levels of Suspicion for Cancer			
	Clinical (P)	Mammography (M)	Ultrasound (U)	Histopathology (B)
1.	Normal	Normal	Normal	Inadequate
2.	Benign	Benign	Benign	Benign
3.	Uncertain	Uncertain	Uncertain	Uncertain malignant potential
4.	Suspicious	Suspicious	Suspicious	Suspicious of malignancy
5.	Malignant	Malignant	Malignant	a. Malignant in situ
				b. Malignant invasive

thoroughly investigated at the diagnostic and treatment stages of care. They also oversee continued surveillance imaging investigations after treatment, routine breast screening, and family history surveillance for high risk women for breast cancer.

- *Consultant oncologist*

The oncologist specializes in the nonsurgical treatment of cancer; they advise the team regarding the predicted benefits or limitations of radiotherapy, chemotherapy, and hormone treatments.

- *Breast care nurse*

Breast care nurses play a key supportive role in the pathway of care for patients undergoing investigations and diagnosis. All patients diagnosed with breast cancer are allocated a member of the breast care nursing team as their key worker to provide ongoing support as required throughout and after the treatment pathway.

- *Histopathologist*

Breast pathologists examine tissue samples under the microscope, including biopsy and surgically excised tissue. This helps to inform diagnosis, treatment options, and the type of drugs breast cancers may be sensitive to.

- *Clinical specialist nurse*

This nurse will have specialist clinical skills, and be able to conduct consultations/clinical examination with women with new symptoms or those being followed after treatment for breast cancer.

- *Research nurse*

The research nurse supports the MDT by flagging potential candidates for clinical trials. They will liaise with the woman, giving information and taking consent for participation on trials.

- *MDT facilitator*

The MDT facilitator prepares the agenda for each meeting and records outcomes. They monitor the progress of a woman's pathway and highlight if any breeches in care are imminent.

Extended members of the team may include but are not limited to:

- Clerical staff
- Mammographer
- Radiographer
- Oncology nurse specialist
- Metastatic breast care nurse
- Theater manager
- Support staff
- Junior medical staff (registrars, etc.)
- Physiotherapists
- Psychologist
- Palliative oncologists

As discussed in Chapter 8, some of the responsibilities described earlier may be undertaken by a variety of appropriately trained health care professionals.

Organization of the Multidisciplinary Team

These meetings should happen on a weekly basis and be a fixed clinical commitment. Adequate resources should be provided and supported by an MDT facilitator.

A record of the meeting, including attendance, should be kept and all discussions/conclusions be clearly documented in the patients' notes. Decisions should be made according to written protocols. MDTs are regulated through an annual peer review process, which ensures adherence to national tumor-specific guidelines with the aim to standardize and improve outcomes of cancer patients.

In general, the meeting will have a named chairperson to ensure discussions are focused and the meeting is kept to time; this may or may not be the same person as the lead service clinician.

What Supports an Effective Multidisciplinary Team?

Factors influencing the effectiveness of the MDT are open lines of communication; adequate available clinical, social and psychologic information for each woman; good attendance by each core member; and a dedicated meeting room with electronic displays to view clinical, radiological, and pathological findings. Quality of discussions can be affected by fatigue, as the ever-increasing caseload causes the meeting to grow longer. This can be managed by scheduling a short break mid-meeting.

Frequent governance and operational meetings are recommended for an MDT to ensure current practice is up to date, any audits or service evaluations can be presented and the overall strategic plan for the unit can be reviewed.

What Is Discussed at Multidisciplinary Team Meetings?

The MDT list for discussion will usually consist of several types of patients, for example: newly diagnosed, postsurgical, oncology, metastatic, and further queries.

The woman's history and clinical presentation will be presented, then the imaging and histopathology will be deliberated to establish correlation. If all findings agree, a decision can be made as to whether treatment is required or if the woman can be discharged. If the findings are discordant, further discussion will take place regarding further investigations, such as repeat biopsy or further imaging.

Once the woman has undergone the first line of treatment, their case is usually bought back to MDT to discuss further management. For example, if a breast cancer was surgically excised, the histopathology would be reported, and a discussion would take place to establish if further treatment with radiotherapy or chemotherapy was appropriate.

Overall, the MDT is an essential part of the woman's journey and it is useful for the mammographer to understand their relevance within this team.

Restructuring of Multidisciplinary Teams

As diagnosis rates increase and cases become more complex, some MDTs have become unmanageable and strategies are being put in place to improve efficiency. A pre-MDT triage meeting is now becoming a popular tool, whereby the MDT list is reviewed by a few personnel a day or two in advance and cases that are not requiring full MDT discussion can be considered. If new cases are found to be benign, if all the results are not ready or a protocoled pathway can be delivered, formal MDT discussion may not be required.

CASE STUDY TO DEMONSTRATE A PATHWAY THROUGH THE MULTIDISCIPLINARY TEAM

- Presentation: a 70-year-old woman presented with lump in the upper outer part of the left breast. No discrete lesion; change in contour of the breast.
- Breast surgeon (or other) consultation and physical examination: Clinically benign with contour change, P2.
- In line with routine protocol, the patient met the mammographer who performed bilateral craniocaudal (CC) and mediolateral oblique (MLO) mammograms (Fig. 14.1):

By using their skills and knowledge of the mammography unit, communication skills, breast anatomy, and positioning technique, the mammographer produces diagnostic mammograms.

The resultant mammogram shows:
- the pectoral muscle down to the level of the nipple
- the nipple in profile
- the inframammary folds are tidy
- the exposure factors are correct
- the images are sharp
- there is slightly less tissue demonstrated on the CC views than the MLO views
- there is a slight fold on the left CC image

Overall this would be considered a good mammogram and will help the RA in their role to characterize and classify the mammographic feature. The RA will compare this examination with previous mammograms, as a new feature in a woman of this age raises the level of suspicion for breast cancer. The RA will use the diagnostic tools on the workstation to review and visualize these features and to draw a conclusion. The density in the left breast is very subtle and difficult to visualize on the MLO view, the trigger for the RA is that the density is new. The abnormality on the CC view is an area that can be easily missed on a badly positioned CC view and in this case that would be relevant in both the historical and the current mammogram. If the area was not included on the previous images, the RA would not perceive the interval change potentially leading to a missed diagnosis.

- The mammograms were reviewed by the RA and reported as follows:

Comparison has been made with a previous imaging of 2017, in the upper outer part of the right breast there is the 27 mm focus of suspicious microcalcification.

In the upper outer part of the left breast there is a diffuse abnormality which is new and measuring at least 38 mm with associated equivocal microcalcification. The features overall are mammographically suspicious.

Both breasts: M4

- The RA requested complementary (additional) views of the right breast that would best help them with the accurate characterization of the mammographic features (Fig. 14.2). In this case to localize, determine the extent of the calcification in the right breast, and establish if there is any underlying feature, such as a mass. This will also help the mammographer in deciding the best approach for a stereotactic guided core biopsy and accurate targeting.

- The RA reported the images:

Additional views confirm suspicious microcalcification in the upper outer right breast, M4

As the woman presented with a lump, it is usual practice for an US to be performed of the palpable area. The RA will also use the mammogram to help guide and direct the US. Most units will routinely scan the axilla on the ipsilateral side for a mammographically suspicious feature. This will establish if the disease has spread to the lymph nodes. This will help the surgeon to plan their surgery.

- The RA proceeded to perform bilateral breast and axilla US scans:

Ultrasound of the right breast shows no abnormality.

Ultrasound of the outer left breast showed diffuse change measuring in excess of 35 mm; it is difficult to see if there is multifocal disease and/or an extensive single lesion but features are consistent with malignancy.

No abnormality seen in the right axilla.

An equivocal node noted in the left axilla.

Summary:

Right—U1, Ax1.

Left—35 mm U5, Ax3.

As the additional views of the right breast suggest calcification as the only significant feature; the normal US scan is concordant and it is appropriate to proceed to stereotactic guided core biopsy. The normal US of the axilla is also in keeping with the mammographic findings: the absence of a mass is suggestive of ductal carcinoma in situ (DCIS) rather than invasive disease but as background breast pattern is fairly dense; an underlying invasive component remains a consideration despite the normal US.

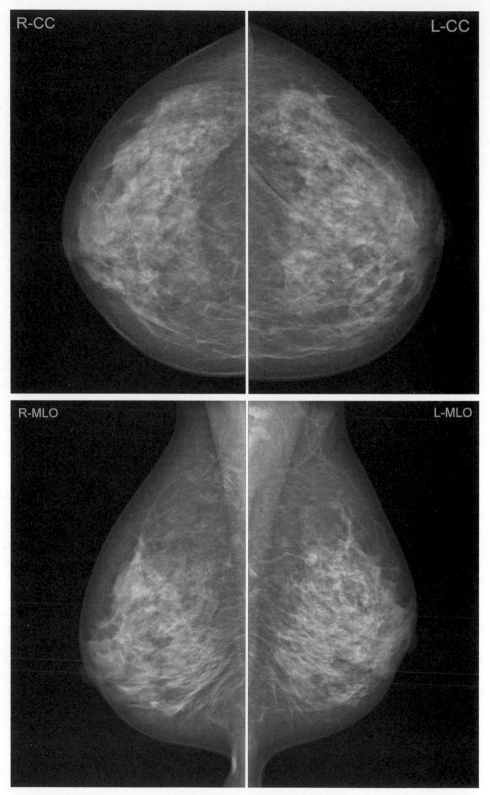

Fig. 14.1 Bilateral craniocaudal *(CC)* and mediolateral oblique *(MLO)* mammograms.

US of the left breast shows the palpable area corresponds with an irregular-shaped solid mass; these are sonographic signs of a malignancy (Fig. 14.3). The RA will correlate this with the mammographic features and the clinical findings. The US features correspond with a new density compared with the previous mammograms of 3 years ago, seen mainly on the CC view. There is a 5-mm focus of calcification in a similar area but although this is likely to be associated, is too small on mammography to represent the extent of the disease, and is unlikely to be palpable. The US abnormality correlates

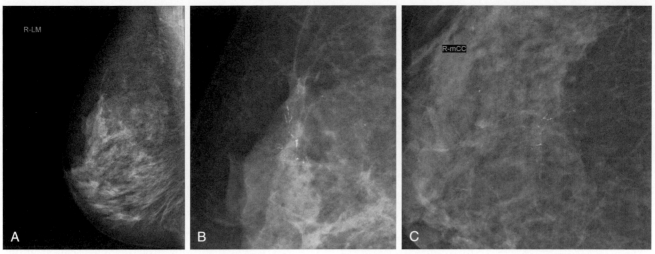

Fig. 14.2 Additional views. (A) Right lateral medial. (B) Right lateral medial magnification. (C) Right craniocaudal magnification.

with the area of concern identified on clinical breast examination; however, there is discordance in the level of suspicion. By combining all of the available information, early indications would suggest a lobular cancer. The axilla scan on the left side showed a single node with some sonographic signs of metastasis.

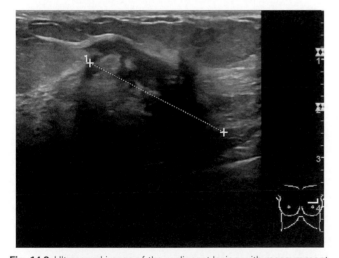

Fig. 14.3 Ultrasound image of the malignant lesion with measurement.

Because the area is most easily seen on US, this was the chosen method for biopsy of the breast and axilla. Correlating the mammographic features with the US findings, the new calcification in the left breast was confirmed as part of the same disease process.

- The RA proceeded to performed US-guided core biopsy of the left breast and axilla with the support of an imaging assistant.

  After discussion with the RA, the mammographer reviews the images to direct the accurate targeting of the calcification in the right breast.
- Stereotactic-guided core biopsy of the calcification in right breast was performed by the RA, with the assistance of a skilled mammographer to adequately position the area of interest (Fig. 14.4).
- Core specimens were imaged to demonstrate representative calcification had been adequately sampled (Fig. 14.5).
- A marker clip was inserted postbiopsy to confirm area sampled (Fig. 14.6). This could also enable US-guided localization if the biopsy was positive for cancer.

  The RA will compare the diagnostic mediolateral view and CC with the postprocedural image to confirm that the clip is correctly sited in relation to the targeted calcification.

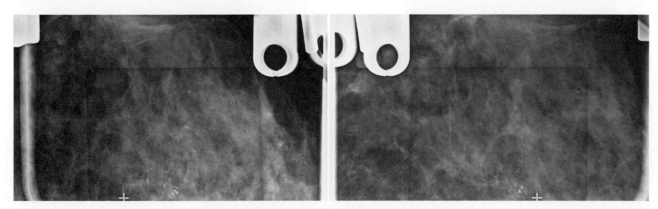

Fig. 14.4 Prebiopsy stereotactic images right breast.

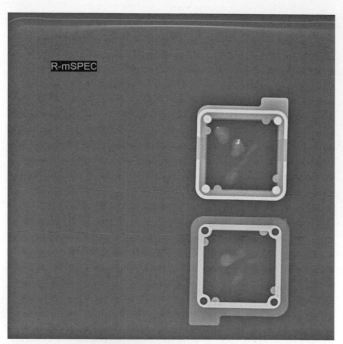

Fig. 14.5 Right magnified x-ray of the core specimens (R-mSPEC) from the stereotactic biopsy.

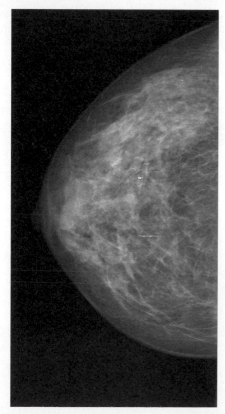

Fig. 14.6 Right mammograms postbiopsy to demonstrate marker clip.

In some cases, there may be no residual calcification and good quality images and accurate tissue marker placement will be important for preoperative localizations.

The core biopsies give a good indication of type of tumor the team are dealing with; this may alter once the whole

lesion has been removed and more tissue is available; this may sometimes lead to further surgery. If there is any discordance, a further biopsy may be indicated before surgery.

- The histopathologist then reported the biopsies as:
  Left breast—invasive lobular carcinoma—B5b
  Left axilla—no evidence of malignancy
  Right breast—invasive ductal carcinoma—B5b
- MDT discussion 1:
  At the MDT, the finding of each specialist will be discussed and correlated. For symptomatic women, the case is usually presented by the surgical team.
  The presenting symptom was a benign feeling nodularity in the upper/outer left breast with change in breast contour. The imaging demonstrated features highly suspicious of malignancy in both breasts. The histopathology was presented showing invasive lobular cancer in the left breast and invasive ductal cancer in the right breast. The team proceeded to discuss the findings and to decide on recommendations for the most appropriate next step.
  The comparative size of the abnormality to the whole breast and the biology of the tumor will help determine the most appropriate management.
  This may be either:
  - a wide local excision (WLE); removal of the cancer from the breast
  - a mastectomy—removal of the whole breast
  - neoadjuvant chemotherapy—chemotherapy before surgery
  Recommendation for the right breast was WLE plus sentinel lymph node biopsy (SLNB). An SLNB is a surgical sample of the nodes in the axilla by identifying with blue dye and or radioisotope the nodes where the tumor is most likely to have spread; this is usually between one and four nodes. Despite US of the right axilla showing normal looking lymph nodes, when invasive malignancy is proven on breast biopsy, it is routine practice to perform surgery in the ipsilateral axilla.
  For the left breast, it was difficult to palpate and size accurately on imaging and the background breast pattern was fairly dense. Because it is difficult to be sure about the extent of the disease and lobular cancer is often multifocal and bilateral, MRI was recommended.
- Summary of MRI report:
  A 25-mm abnormality, corresponding with the known cancer in the right breast, with the marker clip.
  In the left breast there was a 41-mm lesion corresponding with the known cancer. No other suspicious features were seen in either breast, and normal axillary lymph nodes were seen bilaterally.
  Conclusion:
  Right breast-MR5
  Left breast-MR5
- MDT discussion 2:
  The team usually recap on the findings from the original MDT before discussing the new information. The MRI confirms the size and distribution of the known cancers; therefore WLE of both breast cancers with SLNBs are recommended (rather than neoadjuvant chemotherapy or

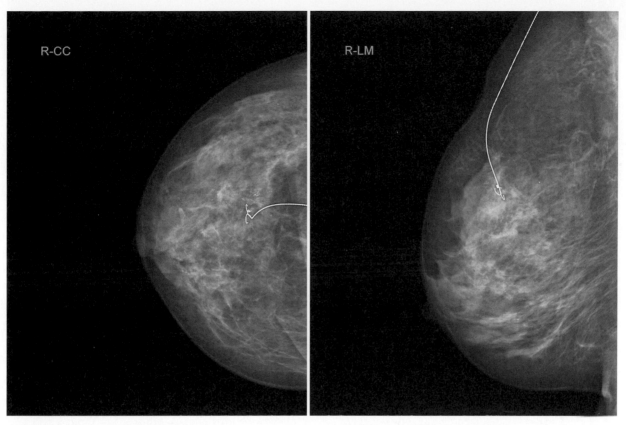

Fig. 14.7 Right craniocaudal (R-CC) and lateral medial (R-LM) post procedure images of right breast demonstrating the wire.

mastectomy). As neither cancer was palpable, they required guide-wire localization and SLNB.

- RA and mammographer perform the localization procedures. They review the diagnostic imaging to accurately target the wire placements. The postprocedure images of the right breast show the wire to be in the expected place in relationship to the marker clip and the residual calcification (Fig. 14.7). The postprocedure images of the left breast show the wire to be within the original new density but the associated calcification is behind the wire (Fig. 14.8). The RA may wish to highlight this to the surgeon as they will need to take this into account during operation.
- The surgeons undertake the operations and image the specimens to evaluate if the lesion has been completely excised at the time of surgery (Figs. 14.9 and 14.10). The calcification within the right breast specimen can be seen extending to the edge; therefore further excision of the relevant margin is indicated. In the left breast specimen, both the density and the associated calcification can be seen, indicating the whole area has been included in the excision.
- Surgical specimens were reported by the histopathologists:
  LEFT breast WLE and SLNB:
  The lesion is a completely excised, 29 mm multifocal Grade 3, invasive lobular carcinoma. No vascular invasion. Widespread LCIS.
  SNLB: At least 2 mm metastases (1/1) with extracapsular spread – spreading beyond the node into the surrounding tissue.

ER positive, PR positive, HER2 negative
RIGHT breast WLE and SLNB:
The lesion was an incompletely excised (lateral margin <1 mm) multifocal pleomorphic grade 2, invasive lobular carcinoma, with solid and cribriform intermediate and high-grade DCIS with comedo necrosis, extending to the lateral margin. Lymphovascular invasion present. Disease is infiltrative and not forming a mass; therefore accurate measurements are not possible, but is approximately 32 mm. The excision of the lateral margin completed a complete excision. SLNB: 1/1 metastatic lymph node with extracapsular spread
ER positive, PR negative, HER2 negative

- MDT discussion 3:
  The team usually recap on the findings from the original MDT before discussing the new information. The surgical histology was discussed in conjunction with the imaging. The histology report will include detailed information to direct the ongoing treatment and prognostic factors for every woman. This will include:
  - The tumor grade: 1 being the least aggressive to 3 the most aggressive
  - Type and subtype: ductal, lobular, basal like
  - Hormone receptor status: estrogen (ER); progesterone (PR)
  - HER2 status: herceptin
  - Nodal status: number of metastatic nodes

All of this information will be useful in deciding the best treatment regime for the individual woman. The pathology

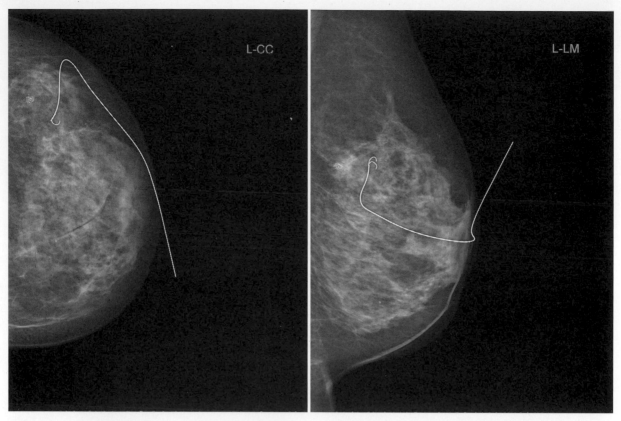

Fig. 14.8 Left craniocaudal (L-CC) and lateral medial (L-LM) post procedure images of left breast demonstrating the wire.

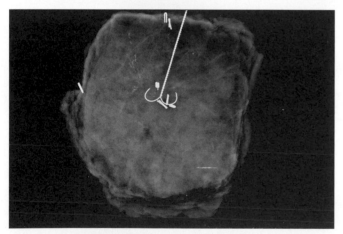

Fig. 14.9 Right breast specimen.

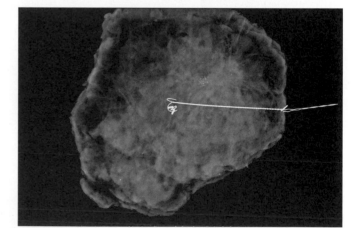

Fig. 14.10 Left breast specimen.

in the right breast altered the invasive tumor type to lobular cancer.

The lesion in the left breast was excised in the original specimen and the right breast lesion was completely excised after taking margins at the time of surgery. Both axillae contained metastatic nodes. All of these factors are taken into consideration when discussing the ongoing management of this woman. The anatomy and biology of the breast and breast cancer will help predict the most effective option. In this case, the oncologist recommended radiotherapy to both breasts and axillae with hormone treatment. Bisphosphonates and systemic therapy were to be discussed.

CONCLUSION OF THE IMPORTANCE OF MULTIDISCIPLINARY TEAMS

Overall, this case study shows how every team member is crucial to both the diagnosis and a personalized management of a woman with breast cancer.

The mammographer will have several interactions with a woman and it is important that she understands the relevance of the quality of care she gives. Optimal image quality is required to inform diagnosis and treatment. A team working approach gives the woman the best possible experience and outcome.

FURTHER READING

Andolina, V., Lille, S. (2011). *Mammographic imaging: a practical guide* (3rd Ed.). Philadelphia: Wolters Kluwer/Lippincott Williams & Wilkins Health.

Bland, K.I., Copeland, E.M., Climber, V.S., Gradishar, W.J. (2017). The breast: comprehensive management of benign and malignant diseases. In *The breast: comprehensive management of benign and malignant diseases.* Elsevier Inc.

Borrelli, C., Cohen, S., Duncan, A., et al (2016). NHSBSP; Clinical guidance for breast cancer screening assessment, publication 49. Public Health England. Available at: https://associationofbreast-surgery.org.uk/media/1414/nhs-bsp-clinical-guidance-for-breast-cancer-screening-assessment.pdf (Accessed 20/04/20).

Gandamihardja, T.A.K., Soukup, T., McInerney, S., Green, J.S.A., Sevdalis, N. (2019). Analysing breast cancer multidisciplinary patient management: a prospective observational evaluation of team clinical decision-making. *World Journal of Surgery,* 43(2), 559–566.

Hogg, P., Kelly, J., Mercer, C. eds (2015). *Digital mammography. A holistic approach.* Switzerland: Springer International Publishing.

Kesson, E.M., Allardice, G.M., George, W.D., Burns, H.J.G., Morrison, D.S. (2012). Effects of multidisciplinary team working on breast cancer survival: Retrospective, comparative, interventional cohort study of 13 722 women. *British Medical Journal (Online),* 344(7856).

Kopans, D.B. (2006). *Breast imaging* (3rd ed). Baltimore, Maryland: Lippincott Williams & Wilkins.

Lee, B., Whitehead, M.T. (2017). Radiology reports: what you think you're saying and what they think you're saying. *Current Problems in Diagnostic Radiology,* 46(3), 186–195.

Maxwell, A.J., Ridley, N.T., Rubin, G., Wallis, M.G., Gilbert, F.J., Michell, M.J. (2009). The Royal College of Radiologists Breast Group breast imaging classification. *Clinical Radiology,* 64(6), 624–627.

National Cancer Peer Review-National Cancer Action Team. (2011). Manual for Cancer Services: Network Service User Partnership Group Measures. Version 1.0. Available at: https://assets.publishing.service.gov.uk/government/uploads/system/uploads/attachment_data/file/216117/dh_125890.pdf (Accessed 21/04/20).

NICE (2002) Improving Outcomes in Breast Cancer. Cancer service guideline [CSG1]. Available at: https://www.nice.org.uk/guidance/csg1 (Accessed 24/04/20).

Public Health England. (2017). NHS Breast Screening Programme Guidance for breast screening mammographers. 3rd Ed. Available at: https://assets.publishing.service.gov.uk/government/uploads/system/uploads/attachment_data/file/819410/NHS_Breast_Screening_Programme_Guidance_for_mammographers_final.pdf (Accessed 16/04/20).

Rajan, S., Foreman, J., Wallis, M.G., Caldas, C., Britton, P. (2013). Multidisciplinary decisions in breast cancer: does the patient receive what the team has recommended? *British Journal of Cancer,* 108(12), 2442–2447.

Shetty, M.K. ed. (2014). Breast Cancer Screening and Diagnosis: A Synopsis. New York: Springer.

Shah, B.A., Fundaro, G.M., Mandava S.R. (2015). *Breast imaging review: a quick guide to essential diagnoses.* 2nd Edition. New York: Springer.

Sibbering, M., Watkins, R., Winstanley, J., Patnick, J. (2009). Quality assurance Guidelines for Surgeons in Breast cancer screening. NHSBSP Publication no 20 fourth edition. NHS Cancer Screening Programmes. Available at: https://assets.publishing.service.gov.uk/government/uploads/system/uploads/attachment_data/file/465694/nhsbsp20.pdf (Accessed 24/04/20).

Sibbering, M. (2020). Improving the efficiency of breast multidisciplinary team meetings: a toolkit for breast services. January Available at: https://associationofbreastsurgery.org.uk/media/251959/breast-mdtm-toolkit-v-3.pdf (Accessed 06/02/20).

Soukup, T., Gandamihardja, T.A.K., McInerney, S., Green, J.S.A., Sevdalis, N. (2019). Do multidisciplinary cancer care teams suffer decision-making fatigue: An observational, longitudinal team improvement study. *British Medical Journal Open,* 9(5), e027303.

Taylor, C., Munro, A.J., Glynne-Jones, R., et al. (2010). Multidisciplinary team working in cancer: what is the evidence? *British Medical Journal,* 340, p.c951.

The Royal College of Radiologists. (2014). *Cancer Multidisciplinary Team Meeting – Standards for Clinical Radiologists.* 2nd edition. Available at: https://www.rcr.ac.uk/sites/default/files/bfcr1415_mdtms_revised_web_final.pdf (Accessed 21/04/20).

The Royal College of Radiologists. (2019). *Guidance on screening and symptomatic breast imaging 4th edition.* November. Clinical Radiology. Available at: https://www.rcr.ac.uk/system/files/publication/field_publication_files/bfcr199-guidance-on-screening-and-symptomatic-breast-imaging.pdf (Accessed 20/04/20).

Wagner, J., Liston, B., Miller, J. (2011). Developing interprofessional communication skills. *Teaching and Learning in Nursing,* 6(3), 97–101.

Wilson, R., Liston, J. (eds) (2011). *Quality Assurance Guidelines for Breast Cancer Screening Radiology.* 59. Sheffield: NHS Cancer Screening Programmes. Available at: https://assets.publishing.service.gov.uk/government/uploads/system/uploads/attachment_data/file/764452/Quality_assurance_guidelines_for_breast_cancer_screening_radiology_updated_Dec_2018.pdf (Accessed 20/04/20).

Page numbers followed by *f* indicates figures and *t* indicates tables.